The Sugar For Therapy Book

By DanM@CowsEatGrass

Disclaimer

The author-publisher, DanM@CowsEatGrass, is not a medical doctor and is not directly or indirectly presenting or recommending any part of this publication's data as a diagnosis or prescription for any medical, psychological, or other ailments of any reader. If anyone uses this information without the advice of their professional health adviser, they are prescribing for themselves, and the author-publisher assumes no responsibility or liability. Persons using any of this data do so at their own risk and must take personal responsibility for what they don't know and what they do know.

The content of this book is not a substitute for advice from a healthcare professional. You should not disregard medical advice or delay seeking it due to opinions, recommendations, or any other information you have read in this book.

The opinions expressed in this book are the opinions of the author. To the extent permitted by applicable law, the author assumes no liability or responsibility for damage or injury to persons or property arising from any use of information, ideas, opinions or instructions found in this book.

Preface

It's not uncommon to hear people talk about sugar issues. Still, they never seem to explain what causes the actual problems that cause "sugar issues". And when causes do get mentioned, it's usually just a bunch of circular arguments blaming sugar, with little concern for logic or biology. So the real villains, the things that promote stress and inflammation and blood sugar dysregulation, get a free pass.

It's one thing to believe sugar isn't that harmful and that it's OK to have some now and then, in moderation. It's different to realise that it is healthy and stress and disease-protective. This book explains why sugar is so good, yet it's easy to believe it isn't. I hope you enjoy it.

You should read this book if the suggestion that sugar is healthy upsets or provokes anger in you or doubt. This book has come from my experimentation with nutrition, years of searching for and reading through biological science, and my interpretation of Dr Ray Peat's work. It is not health advice, and I do not claim it is 100%

correct. I'm not a doctor or a scientist, and I don't expect anybody to follow me or do as I say. And there are no study references included. However, if you want studies, my articles and eBooks are full of them and are available at www.Cowseatgrass.org.

"Let Sugar Be Thy Medicine, and Medicine Be Thy Sugar."

TABLE OF CONTENTS

Introduction

Section A / What Sugar Helps With

Section B / Sugar Stabilises Blood Sugar

Chapter 17 / Stress Causes Blood Sugar Dysregulation

Section C / Digestion, Sugar and Health

Chapter 18 / The Problem With Fasting

Chapter 19 / The Art Of Fasting, Without Fasting

Chapter 20 / Improving Digestion Improves Everything

Section D / Why Quitting Sugar Feels Good

Chapter 21 / Sugar Isn't The Junk In Food

Chapter 22 / Stress Can Feel Good, For a While

Chapter 23 / Hibernation is Not a Lifestyle Choice

Chapter 24 / Not All Sugar Gets Made Equal

Section E / How To Use Sugar Therapeutically

Chapter 25 / Simple Sugar Syrup

Chapter 26 / Sugar Added To Drinks

Chapter 27 / When I Have Sugar

Chapter 28 / How Much Sugar To Use

Chapter 29 / Sugar On Wounds

Section F / Diseases Not Caused By Sugar

Chapter 30 / Autism and Sugar

Chapter 31 / Cancer and Sugar

Chapter 32 / Diabetes and Sugar

Introduction

'The Hatha Yoga Pradipika includes sugar and sugar candy as wholesome foods for the best yogis. Most "yogis" I know think sugar is poison to be avoided, but talk about chia and kale smoothies...' DanM@CowsEatGrass

'Stress seems to be perceived as a need for sugar.' Ray Peat PhD

If you haven't already heard, sugar is medicine. Yes, that's right, I'm talking about plain old white sugar, otherwise known as sucrose. And no, just in case you're wondering, I'm not saying that other foods containing sugar (sucrose, fructose, glucose etc.) aren't healthy healing foods.

There are many healing foods with some sugar in them, which get used to improve health and protect against ill health. I'm also not suggesting that eating sugar and nothing else is a good idea, at least not for too long. But we are here to talk about simple, refined, processed sugar, so I will.

There are a variety of ways that white sugar can be a powerful healing tool. And white sugar is also something that can be highly effective and protective when incorporated into everyday eating. One good reason we're talking about white sugar is that white sugar can be uniquely therapeutic.

White sugar can also be a convenient and easy-to-apply solution, at least partly for many problems. White sugar is one of the cheapest and easiest to access (at least for the time being) regarding high-quality nutrients, energy sources, and medicines; sugar is all three.

It's important to remember that because some say sugar is evil doesn't mean it's true. And it doesn't mean you have to listen. Many people think polyunsaturated fats are healthy; salt causes high blood pressure, milk isn't food for adults, complex carbs are best, and so on.

Do you want to get your health ideas from industry propaganda? I know I don't. However, the fact that you're reading this means that you already know lots of things you got told to eat and take in the past weren't helpful.

Chances are you've already changed your mind about simple sugar, and you're ready to hear some of the great things there are to say about it. So, prepare to listen to a boatload of good stuff about sugar. You're going to love it.

Section A / What Sugar Helps With

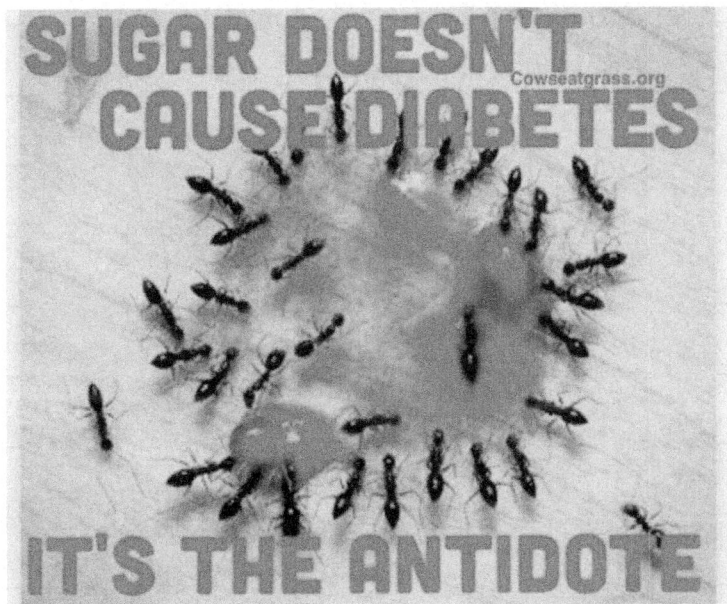

'Once you know what sugar helps with biologically, you know much more about biology than you think. However, you might not know how much you know about biology, so start with sugar and go from there.' Myself

'I'm not here to give you a diet. I'm here to help you distinguish between the truth and the lies. Then you can make up your mind...and create your diet. That's what I do.' CowsEatGrass

After years of exposure to popular dietary advice and "official" recommendations based on questionable science, suggesting that sugar is healthy or even therapeutic naturally sounds radical and unbelievable.

So don't worry if you're still a little sceptical. Who wouldn't be after a lifetime of exposure to one of human history's most extensive psychological operations?

I like to call it the "Let's See If We Can Convince People That Their Number One Source Of Energy Is Responsible For Their Health Problems" plan. I was also considering calling it the "Let's Make Sure People Don't Know How Good Sugar Is, Or We'll Never Be Able To Sell Them Our Poisons" plan.

Anyway, it's a toss-up between those two and some others as well. You get the idea.

Funnily enough, although sugar gets blamed for causing almost every disease under the sun, if you read the science available for everyone, you'll begin to notice something strange. At least I did.

You might realise that all the propaganda pieces keep pushing the "sugar is bad" narrative. Still, the actual biological and medical experiments keep showing the opposite. Of course, there are some exceptions, but after a while, you start to see something wrong with studies that blame sugar for disease. What's wrong is that they often fail to follow the scientific method.

So let's start by examining how sugar is known to benefit from a biological standpoint.

Chapter 1 / Sugar Promotes Thyroid Function>>

The thyroid is at the heart of metabolic energy systems, so whenever we look at metabolic or energy issues, we also look at thyroid-related issues. There's no other way to see it.

To simplify matters, referring to it as the "thyroid energy system metabolism" is not inaccurate. When you suppress thyroid metabolism, energy production is interfered with, reducing the whole organism's performance.

One crucial thing sugar does concerning this is to give the liver fuel, which is necessary to make available a large portion of active thyroid hormone.

You use sugar to convert inactive thyroid hormone (thyroxine T4) into active thyroid hormone (triiodothyronine T3). If you have too much T4 and not enough T3, metabolism will not be optimal. Excess T4 is anti-metabolic. Simple white sugar can provide the energy required to help protect against this kind of imbalance.

Yes, this involves other things simultaneously, but sugar is generally fundamental. And sugar also gives the cell the energy to encourage the conditions required for properly utilising any available thyroid hormone.

A cell under stress, or in other words, a cell without sufficient energy available to meet demand, might not be able to use the thyroid hormone optimally. So this, too, can be powerfully anti-metabolic.

When energy systems are suppressed or interfered with, this increases susceptibility to disease and degeneration. Some illnesses connected to an under-functioning thyroid metabolism include cancer, heart disease, fibromyalgia, arthritis, and autism, to name just a few.

There isn't a disease known to man that isn't, to some degree, related to thyroid issues. So in this sense, sugar is anti-disease, anti-degeneration, and anti-aging.

Unfortunately, however, it isn't just a case of "eat

more sugar, thyroid fixed now" when it comes to improving thyroid energy metabolism. At least not always.

That's not because of anything lacking in the ability of sugar to promote metabolic capability. Instead, because interference with metabolism is cumulative, removing interference with metabolism can require time and several improvements.

But still, there are many excellent reasons why experimenting with increased sugar consumption can make a noticeable positive difference reasonably quickly. And there are several quick and simple ways to test this.

Chapter 2 / Sugar Promotes Cholesterol Production>>

Cholesterol is an anti-stress substance that is fundamental in producing protective, anti-aging, anti-inflammatory substances, pregnenolone, testosterone, progesterone, and DHEA.

Sugar consumption assists in the production of cholesterol. Also, it helps to encourage metabolic conditions, enabling an appropriate level of conversion of cholesterol into protective, more specialised anti-stress substances.

Sugar fuels liver function and the liver is responsible for a large percentage of cholesterol production and thyroid activation.

The thyroid hormone is also required to convert cholesterol into specialised protective substances, including vitamin D and bile. Sugar is essential as a promoter of thyroid, cholesterol, and liver function.

Suppose your blood cholesterol levels are rising. Rather than it being a sign you have too much cholesterol (sneaky cholesterol), it's more likely something is interfering with thyroid energy metabolism.

Stress interferes with thyroid metabolism and is often responsible for the rising demand for cholesterol production. Stress prevents cholesterol from being effectively converted and used for more specialised purposes.

Regarding promoting thyroid metabolism and stress protection, few things are as fundamental as sugar. However, excessive stress and interference with thyroid and cholesterol metabolism interfere with the ability to use sugar properly, so fixing this is rarely as simple as just eating more sugar.

But that's not to say that avoiding sugar is a solution. Instead, incorporating more sugar into your diet to improve metabolism requires understanding how metabolism functions and what interferes with it.

One thing central to thyroid energy system performance is digestion, which needs sugar to function optimally, as much as anything.

Chapter 3 / Sugar Improves Digestion>>

An underactive thyroid metabolism and digestive dysfunction almost always go hand in hand. Digestive issues are very commonly an early sign of metabolic interference. They can play a big part in the slowing of energy systems. Sugar helps by providing the metabolic energy necessary to allow digestion to function faster and more effectively.

Underactive thyroid prominently decreases digestive motility. As digestion slows, toxins build up, partly because of a reduced evacuation speed, leaving waste materials in the system for longer than optimal periods.

By promoting liver function, sugar helps protect against toxins overloading the liver and passing into the system, where they cause more stress and interference with metabolism and damage organ function.

Stress promotes the release of fat from storage to

compensate for the lack of energy provision. Sugar provides the energy required to limit the release of the stress substances that promote this.

By helping to suppress the excessive release of free fatty acids into the blood (which rise when you inhibit metabolism), sugar reduces the quantity of circulating polyunsaturated fats. Polyunsaturated fats (PUFAs) directly interfere with digestion in numerous ways (as well as indirectly via their many thyroid-interfering actions and effects).

The PUFAs interfere with liver function, cholesterol production and conversion, thyroid hormone production, activation, and utilisation. Interference with digestion also directly interferes with liver, thyroid, and cholesterol function.

The PUFAs get promoted as healthy partly because they lower cholesterol levels. Still, they do this not by improving metabolism and cholesterol conversion but by interfering with cholesterol production.

Worse, the PUFAs damage cholesterol, promote inflammation, and powerfully prevent thyroid energy system function, making them anything but good for health. They get marketed as suitable for "fixing" cholesterol issues, but what they're good at is causing the problems that get blamed on cholesterol. These are the same problems that interfere with metabolism and digestion.

An under-functioning digestive system directly increases exposure to many substances that promote stress and inflammation. Still, it also limits the ability to benefit from the food consumed. It creates a vicious circle scenario, and the consumption of easy-to-digest sugar can be uniquely therapeutic under these conditions.

Eating more sugar may not be the answer to every health issue. Still, there are many good reasons to want to ensure that digestion can function well. The sufficient availability of sugar has a vital role to play here.

Poor digestion exacerbates most disease conditions. Excessive stress is synonymous with disease and digestion problems, and digestion problems increase stress. Sugar promotes digestion and lowers stress, so it is safe to say it protects against disease. Sugar is starting to sound good.

Chapter 4 / Sugar Protects Against Stress>>

When stress levels are high, the body goes through glycogen stores much faster than usual. It tends to increase the secretion and circulation of stress-promoting substances, including cortisol and adrenaline.

Excessive stress interferes with digestive function and thyroid metabolism and increases the circulation of polyunsaturated free fatty acids.

Polyunsaturated fats (PUFAs) are anti-metabolic. Therefore, they are preferentially stored away to protect against harm. When sugar availability is inadequate to deal with stress, the stress substances rise to provide alternative fuel. The increased release of fat from storage is one of the first things that happen.

Increased exposure to PUFAs means further suppression of the ability of the cell to produce energy – and use sugar – efficiently. In addition, it means increased exposure to the substances like cortisol and adrenaline, increasing free fatty acid circulation. It is how you create a circular problem.

The liver converts sugar into glycogen, and the more glycogen in storage, the more protection against stress.

Increasing simple sugar consumption can be a fruitful means of preventing or reversing a vicious circle of stress. One way it does this is by keeping glycogen stores well stocked, thereby helping avoid excessive circulation of and exposure to stress substances.

Rising stress substance circulation and increased exposure to PUFAs also interfere with liver function and cholesterol metabolism. Sufficient sugar availability fuels liver function. But it also protects against things that interfere with liver function. It promotes the ability to store increased amounts of glycogen to safeguard against stress for long periods.

As you might already know or are starting to realise, when it comes to metabolic function, all things are interrelated, and all roads lead to sugar.

And because it's difficult to ignore the direct relationship between excessive stress and disease susceptibility, sugar can be your best friend.

Chapter 5 / Sugar Reduces Bacterial Endotoxin Issues>>

When bacteria are allowed to multiply in excess, this increases exposure to endotoxin and other bacterial toxins. There is a direct connection between excess bacteria and bacterial toxins with the onset and development of degenerative diseases, including diabetes, cardiovascular disease, and cancer.

Sugar helps reduce the potential for bacterial issues to escalate in many different ways. Sugar is antibacterial as fueling thyroid energy metabolism improves digestive speed and function, decreasing the opportunity for bacteria to multiply.

A better working metabolism improves intestinal barrier function, which helps prevent bacteria and bacterial endotoxin from entering the primary system. However, increased endotoxin circulation into the main system stresses the liver, directly suppressing thyroid energy system function.

Endotoxin also increases cholesterol requirements and, as such, increases the need for sugar. In addition, rising levels of bacteria and endotoxin in circulation are inflammatory and promote the release of other stress substances that interfere with metabolism.

Endotoxin interferes with blood sugar regulation, and interference with blood sugar is a driver of the stress issues often blamed on sugar consumption. Blood sugar dysregulation increases the release of fat from storage. Free fatty acids (especially PUFAs) interfere with sugar use and promote endotoxin. In addition, the PUFAs worsen intestinal barrier dysfunction, allowing more toxins to pass through to the liver, further inhibiting the ability of the liver to protect against the things that cause stress and inflammation.

Besides protecting against bacterial overgrowth, sugar provides energy to fuel liver function. Improved liver function means improved detoxification of substances that interfere with metabolism. That includes endotoxin, making sugar especially pro-metabolic.

Chapter 6 / Sugar Is An Anti-Serotonin Substance>>

Serotonin secretion in the intestines increases directly in proportion to rising levels of bacterial endotoxin. It is also promoted by increased cortisol levels and other stress-related substances and by releasing polyunsaturated free fatty acids out of storage.

Increased systemic serotonin levels are involved in the processes that result in many disease states and symptoms, including cancer, diabetes and many mental disorders.

Serotonin is anti-thyroid, promotes stress and inflammation, and interferes with liver function. Because thyroid and cholesterol (and the specialised hormones, e.g. progesterone) are the primary protection against harm caused by excess serotonin, sugar plays a fundamental role here.

By fueling digestion and protecting against bacterial endotoxin, sugar reduces serotonin production. In addition, sugar fueling liver function helps remove excess serotonin and helps provide thyroid and cholesterol.

Sugar is anti-serotonin, simply by fueling metabolism. Conversely, rising serotonin directly responds to a lack of metabolic function. Serotonin protects against situations where stress is high, and sugar and other nutrients are insufficiently available. Serotonin reduces metabolic requirements under scarcity, which explains its involvement with hibernation. Although human beings do not hibernate, rising serotonin suppresses metabolic function. And although this is protective in the short term, there are many consequences associated with ongoing exposure to excess serotonin.

Insufficient sugar intake and availability replicate scarcity, and metabolism cannot tell the difference between a famine and a diet. Serotonin slows your system, so you are not entirely eaten away by rising exposure to stress and the substances of stress.

Serotonin closes you down, and sugar opens you

up. In addition, serotonin promotes depression and anxiety, defence mechanisms against excessive demands placed on the system. Unfortunately, ongoing exposure to high serotonin causes many unintended issues, as do chronic depression and anxiety.

The solution to excess serotonin issues is not necessarily only consuming more sugar. Instead, it would help if you considered other things involved with metabolism. However, quitting sugar is not the answer, especially not over the long term.

Many short-term benefits associated with sugar avoidance result from metabolic suppression, reducing symptoms caused by stress and nutritional deficiency. It can be hard to resist, and that's because it can feel like an improvement for a while. Unfortunately, it often takes time for the metabolic damage to become apparent.

The other main reason it seems effective is that when people "quit sugar", they regularly quit many different ingredients. Often these ingredients interfered with digestion and promoted the symptoms caused by endotoxin, serotonin and other stress substances. Eventually, however, stress and suppression of metabolism caused by lack of sugar availability become a bigger problem than what it avoids.

Chapter 7 / Sugar Protects Against Estrogen Dominance>>

Serotonin is a known promoter of the harmful effects of estrogen, and estrogen directly increases serotonin release. In addition, sub-optimal liver function and suppressed thyroid metabolism and digestion promote estrogen excess. Endotoxin and other inflammatory stress substances also promote a rise in estrogen levels.

Estrogen interferes with thyroid function and is a commonly studied cause of cancer. Also, the breakdown products of polyunsaturated fats (PUFAs) magnify the carcinogenic influence of estrogen.

Serotonin, endotoxin, and estrogen are partly responsible for increasing the release of PUFAs from storage as free fatty acids. And by fueling liver function and digestion, sugar encourages the detoxification and excretion of estrogen, powerfully protecting against estrogen dominance.

Sugar consumption can protect against many of the carcinogenic effects of estrogen. It does so by lowering endotoxin and serotonin secretion, promoting thyroid function, stimulating the production of the protective anti-estrogen hormones, reducing free fatty acid release, and simply protecting against the creation of a chronic state of stress and, therefore, estrogen excess.

One theory concerning cancer is that it is a potential response to excessive stress exposure, which causes interference with optimal cellular function. Estrogen is only one of several substances that rise when stress is unmet. Still, one of its fundamental physiological roles is cellular division and multiplication. On the other hand, thyroid hormone and progesterone protect against the impact of estrogen and its excessive buildup in the tissue. And both promote optimal cellular function.

Progesterone requires thyroid and cholesterol metabolism to work correctly, and all three rely on providing energy to make them available in sufficient quantities. The availability of sugar is central to these processes.

Estrogen excess isn't only closely associated with cancer development and spread. There is almost no end to the number of diseases connected to high estrogen exposure levels. This list includes degenerative bone disease, kidney disease, liver disease, thyroid disease, MS, arthritis, diabetes, heart disease, depression, Alzheimer's, and much more.

And it is no coincidence that these conditions also involve suppressed thyroid function and low cholesterol and progesterone supply. In addition, all these disease states involve blood sugar dysregulation. Contrary to popular belief, this is an issue of stress and interference with sugar use, not the result of sugar consumption per se.

The only way to understand how these metabolic issues are related is to know how lack of sugar availability promotes stress and metabolic interference. So again, simply eating more sugar is not necessarily the single-factor solution, but that's not because of anything inadequate about sugar. You need to understand metabolism, and then you can figure out how sugar can be therapeutic.

Chapter 8 / Sugar Protects Against Inflammation>>

Chronic inflammation exists in a large percentage of the diseases of rapid ageing and degeneration. PUFAs and their breakdown products are potent promoters of systemic inflammation.

Other factors that promote inflammation include:

- Rising endotoxin and serotonin circulation.

- Excess estrogen.

- Interference with proper thyroid and digestive function.

A well-fueled energy metabolism protects against stress and reduces the amount of exposure to PUFAs, releasing less into circulation as free fatty acids and keeping inflammation at bay.

Wound healing occurs faster and with less

inflammation when energy systems run well. It is one of the reasons why sugar has proven to be so effective for healing potentially dangerous open wounds. Unfortunately, people with diabetes have problems with healing. However, understanding diabetes as an energy system disorder related to stress and inflammation helps explain why sugar can effectively heal diabetic ulcers. Therefore, the idea that sugar causes diabetes but promotes the healing of diabetic wounds is less than logical.

Stress and suppressed metabolism increase bacterial endotoxin, which irritates the intestines, causing a rise in serotonin. Serotonin is anti-metabolic pro-stress and promotes an increase in the release of PUFAs and interference with the intestinal barrier. It allows more of the inflammatory things to pass through to the liver, overloading it and letting more into circulation in the primary system. Serotonin and endotoxin both increase inflammation. Fueling metabolism and lowering stress with sugar can help protect against all of the above.

Cholesterol is anti-inflammatory and converts into highly protective, inflammation-reducing hormones. It includes pregnenolone and progesterone. Cholesterol also protects against increasing levels of endotoxin and other toxins.

Sugar increases cholesterol production and conversion.

Pregnenolone and progesterone also protect against estrogen dominance. Excess estrogen is anti-metabolic and inflammatory.

The breakdown products of the PUFAs damage cholesterol and allow estrogen and other stress substances to cause more inflammation and disease. Estrogen also interferes with proper wound healing, and thyroid hormone helps heal wounds. None of this is by coincidence.

So sugar again provides the fuel necessary to help reduce many interrelated issues. For example, sugar encourages a well-functioning and robust metabolism, reducing exposure to the mediators of inflammation and limiting the progression of chronic inflammatory disease states. Most people know that excessive or ongoing inflammation advances almost every disease state.

Chronic inflammation is well known to drive the growth and spread of cancer. Not by accident, all things that protect against inflammation also protect against cancer. There is no reason for sugar to be an exception.

Chapter 9 / Sugar Improves Mood>>

Sugar provides the energy the brain requires to function at an optimal level. The more stress a person gets exposed to, the more energy the brain needs to perform well. It can directly impact mood and the progression of mental disorders.

When stress is high, and the energy supply is inadequate, the stress substances – cortisol, adrenaline, estrogen, serotonin, etc. – rise. These and other stress-promoting inflammatory things play a role in the progression of psychological dysfunction.

Evidence supports the idea that chronic and excessive exposure to inflammation promotes, maybe even causes, the so-called disorders of the mind. And there is also a large body of work demonstrating the relationship between depression and anxiety, as well as schizophrenia and PTSD, with high levels of stress hormones, particularly cortisol, estrogen, and serotonin.

Even bacterial endotoxin is a factor in the development of mental distress. And as already stated, all of these things are interrelated and directly result from interference with thyroid energy systems. So it isn't wrong to see depression and anxiety as insufficient energy.

It is a well-known fact that there is a direct link between digestive distress and state of mind. Digestion issues can cause mental dysregulation, and psychological and emotional stress often impacts the digestive system. Most people are aware of this from experience.

The stress substances interfere with digestion, and exposure to the stress substances rises when you inhibit digestion. Poor digestion promotes bacterial endotoxin exposure. Cholesterol increases to help deal with endotoxin issues, and sugar stimulates the production of cholesterol. Low cholesterol worsens the severity of depression and related issues, increasing the likelihood of accidents, violence and suicide.

Increased exposure to PUFAs due to stress and lack of sugar availability promotes inflammation, stress substance release, and digestive interference. And rising exposure to the PUFAs and their breakdown products are directly connected with the rising severity of depression, anxiety, PTSD and schizophrenia.

And what can help with all of the above? You know what I will say, but I'll say it anyway. It's sugar. And before you ask, no, I'm not saying that all you need to do is eat more sugar, and all your problems will miraculously disappear, not every time, at least.

Chapter 10 / Sugar Improves Fat Composition>>

PUFAs and their breakdown products are a significant factor in promoting inflammation and disease. The body prefers not to use them, so they are preferentially stored away. As a result, they build up in tissue over time.

If you're wondering what happens to sugar if you ever eat more than your system can use or store as glycogen, wonder no more. It gets converted into fat and eventually placed into storage for later use. But not just any fat. It doesn't get made into the inflammatory PUFAs, and that's for a good reason. The body knows what it is doing.

Excess sugar, which cannot be used or stored as glycogen, will be primarily converted into mono and saturated fats. These fats are anti-inflammatory and pro-metabolic. So any excess sugar converted into fat this way will assist in moving fat stores away from a high composition of PUFAs, thereby protecting against future interference with metabolism.

And it's important to note that PUFAs play a significant role in developing blood sugar-related issues, such as insulin resistance, interfering with the ability to use sugar optimally. So can you see how eating sugar helps fix the problems that prevent proper sugar use, which, unfortunately, are blamed on overeating sugar?

Changing the body's fat composition away from excess PUFAs also protects against excessive exposure to endotoxin, cortisol, estrogen, and serotonin. And fewer PUFAs in circulation also protect against damage to cholesterol. Oxidised damaged cholesterol is involved in many of the issues incorrectly blamed on cholesterol per se concerning inflammatory conditions, particularly heart disease.

PUFAs play a big part in causing interference with the thyroid in general. So, it's possible to see how sugar, if it helps to improve overall fat composition, is pro-metabolic and anti-disease.

Can you overeat sugar and, as a result, turn sugar into fat in large amounts and put it in the wrong places, causing problems? The short answer is yes, but it's more complicated than many think. And it occurs because of a combination of factors interfering with metabolism. But sugar gets the blame.

When you damage a system so it can no longer metabolise sugar properly, sugar isn't responsible for what happens when you eat it. And taking sugar out of the diet won't fix those issues. However, going slow when reintroducing sugar might be necessary after years of stress and sugar avoidance.

Remember, things referred to as sugar aren't always made of sugar entirely, or in some instances, at all.

Chapter 11 / Sugar Helps Build And Maintain Muscle>>

It's known that chronically high stress and excessive cortisol exposure eat through muscle tissue, sometimes very rapidly. It's also known that ongoing inflammation damages muscles and other vital tissue.

Lack of sugar signals cortisol release, for the apparent purpose of providing the sugar necessary for survival, via eating through (converting) muscle tissue and protein consumed in the diet.

Thyroid suppression is also well understood to promote muscle dysfunction of wide varieties. Most people with thyroid-related issues mention muscular symptoms (stiffness, myalgias, cramps, easy fatigability). None of this will surprise you as you start to work out the interrelated ways our biological systems work.

Are excess serotonin, estrogen, and bacterial endotoxin, also factors playing a role in muscle issues? Yes. Serotonin syndrome is a good example. Severe muscle spasms and tissue breakdown is well known to occur.

Estrogen has a fundamental physiological role in muscle growth, but excess exposure to estrogen damages muscle. Menopause is associated with increased visceral fat mass and decreases in bone mass density, muscle mass, and strength. It is popular to think of menopause as an estrogen-deficient condition. But estrogen levels rise in the tissue post-menopause, which does not appear in estrogen blood tests.

On top of this, progesterone levels decline significantly. As a result, it causes an increase in unopposed estrogen, promoting inflammation and metabolic stress. In addition, the buildup of PUFAs in storage fosters the production of estrogen inside fat cells, which worsens interference with thyroid metabolism and harms muscle tissue.

Approximately half of all patients with cancer eventually develop a syndrome of cachexia, with anorexia and a progressive loss of adipose tissue and muscle mass. The loss of skeletal muscle is the most apparent symptom of cancer cachexia, but cardiac muscle also gets depleted. It is responsible for the death of approximately a quarter of cancer patients.

Cachexia also gets seen in other medical conditions, including AIDS, chronic obstructive pulmonary disease, multiple sclerosis, chronic heart failure, and tuberculosis. Systemic inflammation, as is increased serotonin levels, is a hallmark of cancer cachexia. Cachexia is a high-stress, suppressed thyroid metabolism catabolic state. It makes sense that all the things that protect against excessive stress are likely protective, and sugar is no exception.

Stress and lack of sugar availability increase the circulation of the PUFAs, promoting inflammation and oxidative damage. And there is a known detrimental association between the breakdown products of PUFAs and muscle strength and early muscle wasting among post-stroke patients. A byproduct of the breakdown of PUFAs, malondialdehyde, gets used as a biomarker of muscle weakness and wasting in post-stroke patients.

What about endotoxin? Have a look into sepsis and severe muscle wasting. None of this is coincidental. It's basic biology. But you have to look at the big picture of biology to see how things interrelate. For example, sugar promotes thyroid function and the production of protective substances, including progesterone. Cholesterol and thyroid are the main ingredients for the production of progesterone. Muscle pain and weakness are frequent complaints in people taking cholesterol-lowering medication.

Sugar promotes cholesterol production and metabolism. Cholesterol protects against excess endotoxin and is a primary anti-stress anti-inflammation substance. So sugar protects muscle in a multitude of ways. How do I love thee sugar?

And to add a cherry on top, as I mentioned earlier, sugar helps you get the maximum benefit from the protein you eat. How nice.

Chapter 12 / Sugar Improves Brain Function>>

When the inflammatory substances that rise under stress interfere with energy systems, this can result in a general state of cellular excitation, encouraging the progression of various degenerative brain disorders.

The brain requires a lot of sugar to carry out its many vital functions (including the production of steroid hormones). As stress and brain activity increase, energy or sugar requirements also rise.

Insufficient sugar availability under stress can promote a vicious circle of rising stress substances. Free fatty acids (PUFAs), estrogen, cortisol, endotoxin and serotonin get included, all of which can interfere with brain function.

And stress and the things that rise under stress can

prevent the brain from being able to utilise the sugar made available optimally. It's known that in Alzheimer's disease, there are elevated endotoxin levels in the blood and brain. The breakdown products of the PUFAs are also directly involved in Alzheimer's.

Alzheimer's now gets referred to as "type 3 diabetes", and that's not because it's caused by eating sugar. However, many have misinterpreted scientific results to suggest that. Blood sugar dysregulation and energy dysfunction are related to sugar, of course. But they aren't caused by sugar, a crucial difference many people miss.

Look into the science, and you'll see evidence that "sugar issues" (including the various issues of hypometabolism in the brain, like Alzheimer's) are caused to a large degree by the byproducts and promoters of stress and inflammation. That means the breakdown products of PUFAs (including fish oil), endotoxin, cortisol, estrogen, serotonin, and other inflammatory things that I have yet to mention. In addition, of course, iron dysregulation is an important one. Endotoxin alone is a significant driver of neuroinflammation and neurodegeneration.

Once again, we realise that sugar is protective and

therapeutic because it lowers stress and fuels thyroid energy metabolism. But of course, that's not to say that you can eat more sugar and make years of cumulative damage to metabolic systems immediately disappear.

Getting the full therapeutic benefits from increased sugar consumption can take time, experimentation, and understanding the many things that interfere with thyroid energy metabolism. However, that does not detract from the importance of sugar. And it does not preclude the possibility that the consumption of simple white sugar can be the thing that makes the difference required to allow for healing.

Chapter 13 / Sugar Regulates Immune System Function>>

You don't need to look far to find information about the relationship between the immune system and thyroid metabolism. Some people blame immune issues as the cause of many thyroid issues. Conversely, some argue that thyroid suppression promotes immune dysregulation.

However you look at it, it's evident that they are interrelated issues. So improving thyroid energy metabolism protects you in a way that limits the requirement for overactivation of the immune system. Similarly, improving metabolism reduces the need for exposure to inflammation. Can you see how sugar can be an essential element in this story?

Endotoxin circulating in the system is a potent activator of the immune system, so keeping the digestive system and the liver functioning more optimally is highly important regarding immune regulation.

And cholesterol protects against endotoxin and inflammation, as do the protective hormones made from cholesterol and thyroid hormones. As stated earlier, sugar fuels metabolism, liver function, digestion, and cholesterol production and conversion, so these are good reasons to love sugar.

Of course, remember the breakdown products of PUFAs. The breakdown of PUFAs is called lipid peroxidation. It activates the immune system in the pathogenesis of alcoholic liver disease. Malondialdehyde (MDA), 4-hydroxynonenal (HNE), and acrolein are some breakdown products of seed oils and fish oil that contribute. And there are many other examples available. Evidence shows that lipid peroxidation-related antibodies are present with nonalcoholic fatty liver disease (NAFLD) and are associated with advanced fibrosis. In addition, the breakdown of PUFAs strongly correlates with lupus disease-associated antibody levels.

The metabolism-suppressing and immunosuppressive effects of fish oil or fish oil byproducts get misinterpreted. Fish oil consumption can temporarily reduce symptoms, including inflammation, which many see as a sign of genuine anti-inflammatory thyroid improvement. However, it is a form of suppression of metabolism and immune system function. It is closely tied together and associated with the progression of degenerative diseases, including cancer. Fish oil also makes immune system T-cells vulnerable to bacterial infection. In addition, it can directly interfere with the immune system's ability to deal with viruses and cancer cells.

The breakdown products of the PUFAs interfere with the ability to use sugar. They can detract from the protective and therapeutic role of sugar. However, avoiding sugar increases stress and exposure to PUFAs, and it is certainly not the solution to this problem. The combination of limiting the inflammatory thyroid-suppressive things, especially PUFAs, with increased sugar intake can lead to significant improvement in immune system function.

Chapter 14 / Sugar Lowers Lactic Acid>>

Lactic acid (or lactate) rises under stress and mimics stress. Lactic acid increases when the thyroid is suppressed and interferes with thyroid function. Lactic acid rises when sugar metabolism is interfered with, and lactic acid inhibits the use of sugar. Lactic acid promotes inflammation, and inflammation promotes lactic acid. Lactic acid is a powerful promoter of stress and disease.

The breakdown products of the PUFAs promote the production of lactic acid, and lactic acid stimulates the release of PUFAs into circulation as free fatty acids. Sugar deprivation encourages the production of lactic acid.

Lactic acid places the liver under additional stress. Lactic acid also directly contributes to cancer growth and spread, and high levels are associated with poor clinical outcomes. In cachexia patients, converting glucose to lactic acid (the Cori cycle) accounts for around 50% of total glucose turnover, compared to 20% in cancer patients with stable weight. In addition, lactic acid promotes inflammation, which drives cachexia, and many other diseases incorrectly blamed on sugar.

Endotoxin, which also causes inflammation, promotes cancer and increases lactic acid. And developing lactic acidosis in septic patients is considered an ominous event.

When sugar cannot get used effectively, this increases lactic acid production. Still, once again, sugar per se is not responsible for the inability to properly use sugar. It can be unclear at first. However, once you get your head around it, you will see that sugar deprivation exposes you to everything responsible for an inability to metabolise sugar properly. It includes increased lactic acid. Also, polyunsaturated free fatty acids have a significant role to play.

By lowering exposure to stress substances and promoting thyroid energy production, cholesterol production, and digestive and liver function, sugar protects against endotoxin, excess lactic acid production and more. Sugar sounds impressive.

Chapter 15 / Sugar Reduces Nitric Oxide Exposure>>

Contrary to popular mythology, increasing nitric oxide levels is not good. But, in small amounts to help protect against local stress or thyroid insufficiency, it is a good thing as a backup safety mechanism. Like most stress substances, it does have a vital role.

But rising systemic levels of nitric oxide go hand in hand with disease and inflammation. As a result, they often end up being one of the main factors worsening metabolism.

You produce nitric oxide in response to interference with cellular energy production. It blocks the mitochondria's key respiratory enzyme (cytochrome c oxidase). As a result, it prevents the use of oxygen by the cell. And what does that do? It interferes with energy production. Can you see the problem? Interference with energy production promotes stress. And then stress messes with energy metabolism.

So then, you produce more of the stress substances that inhibited energy production in the first place.

And now you have more stress, which further inhibits energy production. So it can turn into a downward spiralling vicious circle.

Everything that encourages thyroid/oxidative energy metabolism limits stress and protects against excess nitric oxide, and everything that promotes nitric oxide suppresses the thyroid.

Increased exposure to by-products of the highly unstable PUFAs, and rising nitric oxide levels, go together, and both directly prevent optimal energy production. When energy production is interfered with, you inhibit digestion. Bacterial issues then become a problem in the intestines, increasing endotoxin release. Low energy, endotoxin, PUFAs and nitric oxide have a significant role in sepsis.

Suppressed thyroid energy metabolism and high stress allow bacterial endotoxin to enter the primary system. The endotoxin directly interferes with energy metabolism, causes inflammation, and increases nitric oxide wherever it lands.

Increased endotoxin circulation and the by-products of the PUFAs interfere with liver function. In addition, this causes systemic levels of estrogen and serotonin to rise. Both estrogen and serotonin suppress cellular energy metabolism and increase stress, causing nitric oxide to rise. Nitric oxide also promotes prostaglandin production, which increases inflammation. These combinations can lead to severe issues.

The stress substances can over-excite and irritate cells, increasing lactic acid production, lowering CO_2 levels, and inhibiting the use of sugar and oxygen. All this promotes more nitric oxide and encourages "cancer metabolism", where cells can only divide and multiply.

Nitric oxide also increases growth hormone, which causes a more significant release of PUFAs out of storage. Growth hormone interferes with intestinal barrier function, increasing exposure to endotoxin and serotonin. It promotes estrogen and raises nitric oxide levels significantly. Together with these things, growth hormone drives inflammatory disease, particularly cancer.

Excess stress promotes nitric oxide, central to developing and spreading every metabolic stress disease. It also inhibits every process for protection against disease.

Nitric oxide interferes with insulin production, promotes insulin resistance, and thickens and hardens blood vessels and arteries. It damages heart function, prevents oxygen use, and breaks DNA strands. In addition, it interferes with testosterone and progesterone production. It promotes estrogen, serotonin, lactic acid, endotoxin and histamine excess.

It's tempting to want to blame sugar for this. However, it should be more evident to you now that talking about the harm caused by sugar refers to the damage caused by interference with sugar. It is also known as excess stress.

So from that perspective, you don't want to try fixing your health by quitting sugar, and you don't want to try restoring your health by raising nitric oxide levels. But on the other hand, sugar protects against stress and excess nitric oxide and improves health.

Chapter 16 / Sugar Promotes Carbon Dioxide>>

Increased carbon dioxide production and retention is the opposite of high lactic acid and nitric oxide. Another way to say that is that carbon dioxide increases with improved thyroid energy metabolism.

So carbon dioxide levels rise as sugar gets used better for fuel. The reverse is also true. Increased carbon dioxide means improved utilisation of sugar for energy.

As stress substance exposure goes down, carbon dioxide (CO_2) levels increase; increasing CO_2 lowers stress. An easier way to explain it is to say that a high CO_2 state (within safe limits) is a low-stress state.

CO_2 is anti-stress, and sugar is pro-CO_2.

Anything that interferes with thyroid energy system function can hinder the ability of the body to produce CO_2, eventually lowering overall metabolic performance. In addition, stress promotes hyperventilation (or over-breathing), and hyperventilation promotes stress, low CO_2, and interference with metabolism.

Excess stress and the chronic suppression of thyroid energy metabolism promote many diseases. Part of this is the critical link between suppressed thyroid, hyperventilation, and low CO_2 levels in the body. Also, as energy systems are interfered with, and CO_2 decreases, lactic acid production tends to rise. As you already know, increasing exposure to lactic acid is another important factor in disease promotion.

The presence of CO_2 is a good indicator of effective mitochondrial energy production. When stress or thyroid dysfunction interferes with this process, cells produce energy less effectively. They shift to a less efficient state, increasingly converting glucose to lactic acid (rather than CO_2). As a result, they rely more upon fat oxidation for energy, much of which (particularly these days) tends to be polyunsaturated fatty acids (PUFAs).

Thyroid hormone availability and functionality are central to oxidative metabolism and CO_2 production. PUFAs interfere with thyroid hormones on many physiological levels.

The hypothyroid hyperventilation state promotes adrenaline and cortisol. It further interferes with mitochondrial respiration, inhibiting thyroid function, shifting towards fat oxidation, decreasing CO_2 and increasing lactic acid. And lactic acid interferes with metabolism and causes more stress.

Lactic acid production can become chronically increased due to continuous metabolic interference. It can make it more challenging to return to optimal function (with effective glucose oxidation and CO_2 production). Metabolic suppression, hyperventilation, and low CO_2 promote hypoxia, which is central to cancer progression.

Stress and suppressed metabolism promote the absorption into circulation of bacterial endotoxin, further damaging respiration and increasing the release of many stress-related substances (such as serotonin, estrogen and nitric oxide), which can cause more stress, inflammation, and interference with energy metabolism.

Hyperventilation, low CO_2, and rising serotonin and nitric oxide levels are involved in worsening asthma severity. In addition, there is a relationship between asthma and mood disorders like depression or anxiety, also known as hypometabolic stress conditions.

There is an increased risk of cancer among patients with severe asthma. And there is a connection between cancer, anxiety, and depression. So increased CO_2 (and decreased lactate) production is likely protective.

CO_2 lowers exposure to lactic acid and other stress hormones, PUFAs and endotoxin, improving thyroid energy production. It further increases CO_2 production, reducing stress even more.

Sugar helps in many ways because low sugar interferes with thyroid hormone production. It reduces CO_2, moves things toward stress and inflammation, and away from efficient oxidative energy production.

The high lactic acid in the blood is a primary sign of stress and chronic inflammation and an indication of suppressed thyroid. Therefore, anything that promotes oxidative metabolism and reduces lactic acid is protective against disease, and CO_2 is a pro-metabolism, anti-stress, and anti-inflammatory substance.

Chronic metabolic stress, thyroid dysfunction, and inflammation are all related to the development of cancer, heart disease, and diabetes, as well as conditions such as asthma, depression, and anxiety. Conversely, improving metabolism and CO_2 production helps to lower lactic acid, estrogen, serotonin, nitric oxide, free fatty acids, and other inflammatory disease-promoting things.

The things that get a bad name today, including sugar, salt, CO_2, saturated fats, cholesterol, testosterone, and progesterone, are protective. Conversely, the things that can be the most harmful, like estrogen, serotonin, nitric oxide, lactic acid, PUFAs, and iron, get a free pass. Who knows why?

Section B / Sugar Stabilises Blood Sugar

If you think sugar is harmful now... wait till you see what it does when you stop eating it.

CowsEatGrass.org

'It's perfectly understandable for it to appear as self-evident that sugar restriction will lower blood sugar levels. Many see this – so-called improvement in the symptoms of diabetes – as representative of metabolic recovery.'
Blood Sugar Beliefs, CowsEatGrass

Many things can impact blood sugar (and not all of them are harmful). Still, excessive stress leads to hyperglycemia, hypoglycemia, and insulin resistance.

And we all know (well, some of us do anyway) that stress can be alleviated by sucrose and other kinds of sugar in the diet, not by avoiding sugar.

Quitting sugar might feel right for a while. You might even think it's suitable for blood sugar regulation purposes. But the reasons you believe that are easily explained and have nothing to do with sugar being bad per se.

I discuss some reasons for the confusion in Section D, Why Quitting Sugar Feels Good. But for now, let's examine how sugar helps with blood sugar dysregulation issues.

Chapter 17 / Stress Causes Blood Sugar Dysregulation>>

'Removing white "processed" sugar from the diet has been made to sound appealing as a simple solution to blood sugar dysregulation issues and related metabolic problems. There are several biologically logical reasons to avoid that trap.' Cows

When sugar is restricted and you deplete glycogen stores, the stress hormones cortisol and adrenaline rise. It is an attempt to maintain the supply of blood sugar and make available alternative fuel in the form of free fatty acids from storage.

Cortisol maintains blood sugar – partly by blocking the use of sugar for many purposes (e.g.

immune cell function) and converting valuable muscle and other tissue into fuel for cells.

Suppose free fatty acids are high in polyunsaturated fats (PUFAs). In that case, they can lead to a chronic inability of cells to use glucose, leading to chronic hyperglycemia and the release of cortisol. The breakdown products of PUFAs stimulate cortisol synthesis directly. They are closely associated with the progression and severity of the blood sugar dysregulation symptoms that lead to type 2 diabetes.

Adrenaline, cortisol, and PUFAs promote insulin resistance, and insulin resistance encourages blood sugar instability. And starches, or complex carbohydrates, especially when combined with PUFAs, can rapidly raise blood sugar because they quickly convert to pure glucose. It is not to say that starches are terrible, and to avoid them. It is, however, something to keep in mind when healing metabolic dysregulation issues. How a person does with starch depends to some degree on individual digestive/metabolic conditions (and the source of starch). Still, the fact that starches can rapidly raise glucose and powerfully stimulate insulin can cause issues, including increased fat storage. In addition, indigestible starches are problematic for other reasons, particularly concerning the promotion of bacterial overgrowth.

Excess insulin can exacerbate blood sugar issues. The hypoglycemic effects of insulin promote cortisol, adrenaline, and the release of PUFAs. As a result, it can lead to hyperglycemia and excessive fat production. Conversely, chronically raised insulin or insulin resistance promotes stress, and sugar or sucrose is anti-stress.

The fructose component of sucrose slows the rate at which the glucose component enters the bloodstream, reducing the insulinogenic effect of glucose. And insulin is not required to metabolise fructose. In addition, fructose promotes the replenishment of glycogen stores, which protects against stress.

Low sugar availability (and high cortisol) impacts metabolic conditions in various ways, including interference with thyroid function and promoting the harmful effects of the stress substances (like serotonin and endotoxin), driving numerous inflammatory factors.

These stressful, inflammatory conditions interfere with the use of sugar for energy production and can promote illness progression, including obesity. In addition, suppressed thyroid and slow digestion can mean undercooked, hard-to-digest starches are more likely to become food for bacteria.

High-fat diets (high in PUFAs in particular) interfere with thyroid energy systems, which slows liver function. And a damaged liver promotes low blood sugar and stress, increasing exposure to cortisol and adrenaline and releasing PUFAs out of storage, further interfering with blood sugar regulation.

Thyroid dysfunction also inhibits digestion and intestinal barrier function, increasing bacterial issues. Bacterial excess means more endotoxin. And then endotoxin (LPS) promotes hyperglycemia and insulin resistance. And a high-fat meal, in general, can increase systemic endotoxin circulation.

PUFAs and their breakdown products are potent drivers of blood sugar dysregulation. Evidence shows that they reduce the ability of cells to use glucose, causing an increase in cortisol. And PUFAs promote stress substances like serotonin and estrogen. In addition, they increase free radicals, cytokines, and prostaglandins, causing inflammation. As a result, PUFAs encourage many kinds of inflammatory diseases, including diabetes and cancer.

PUFAs disturb many cellular functions, directly interfering with metabolic energy production by damaging the oxidising ability of the cell. Suppression of energy production can increase oxidative (or reductive) stress. Sugar often gets blamed for these issues, but sugar consumption per se is not responsible for this. As mentioned earlier, sugar protects against exposure to PUFAs in various ways. One way is by promoting thyroid energy metabolism.

The saturated fats can also protect against some of the damaging effects of the PUFAs, helping to limit stress and inflammation caused by PUFAs and their breakdown products. Fortunately, excess sugar can promote the production of saturated fats, protecting thyroid metabolism.

Quitting sugar promotes thyroid dysfunction. The relationship between metabolic stress and lack of sugar is well known, as is the relationship between PUFAs and inflammatory stress. A consistently low sugar supply often means cortisol stays high, and PUFAs circulation becomes problematic. It can lead to chronic liver issues, inflammation, digestive distress and difficulty returning to optimal function.

Suppressing thyroid energy systems, liver issues, and increased bacterial endotoxin circulation raises stress substances, including estrogen, serotonin, nitric oxide, and lactate. And stress substances are associated with blood sugar dysregulation.

Many of the things blamed on sugar consumption result from high lactic acid. For example, there is a relationship between increased lactic acid production, diabetes, and cancer progression. PUFAs interfere with oxidative metabolism, lowering CO_2 and promoting lactic acid production, but this gets ignored in favour of a sugar-demonising ideology. Awareness of sugar restriction's impact on lactic acid, inflammation, and disease is often shocking.

Reducing stress and improving thyroid/oxidative metabolism improves function reducing reliance on stress systems. Another way to say this is that sugar is a primary anti-stress pro-thyroid substance.

Sugar also assists with the production of cholesterol and the conversion of cholesterol into anti-inflammatory protective hormones. These include pregnenolone, progesterone, testosterone, and DHEA. They all protect against blood sugar dysregulation symptoms.

Sugar protects against thyroid energy dysfunction, liver issues, and bacterial endotoxin excess. In addition, it helps with cortisol, adrenaline, estrogen, serotonin, nitric oxide, lactate and free fatty acid excess. It prevents cholesterol, pregnenolone, progesterone, testosterone, and DHEA deficiency. So that's many things biology has shown to be involved in blood sugar dysregulation.

People often associate junk food with sugar. But the truth about most "junk food" is that it gets filled with harmful ingredients. Some have very little white sugar or sucrose in them at all. Instead, it is customary to find large quantities of PUFAs, many types of chemicals and preservatives, various unhealthy gums, heavy metals, and other potentially harmful and stressful things.

Often all carbohydrates get lumped together as high in sugar. But grains, for example, are also a source of PUFAs and other anti-metabolic things. In addition, many grains promote bacterial overgrowth, increasing endotoxin exposure, interfering with metabolism and causing stress, inflammation and blood sugar issues. So there can be many benefits to removing grains from the diet.

Still, it is misleading to suggest that this is because of the removal of sugar.

Removing sugar from the diet can sometimes create the illusion of improving blood sugar regulation issues by temporarily lowering readings and giving a false impression of health improvement by suppressing metabolic requirements. But this kind of symptom suppression is only temporary.

Stress causes blood sugar dysregulation, and sugar protects against stress. So that means sugar protects against blood sugar dysregulation.

Whenever sugar seems unable to help or seems like it is making things worse, make sure you look to see where the stress is because I guarantee it will be there somewhere.

I think you know how the saying goes, "follow the stress".

Section C /
Digestion, Sugar and Health

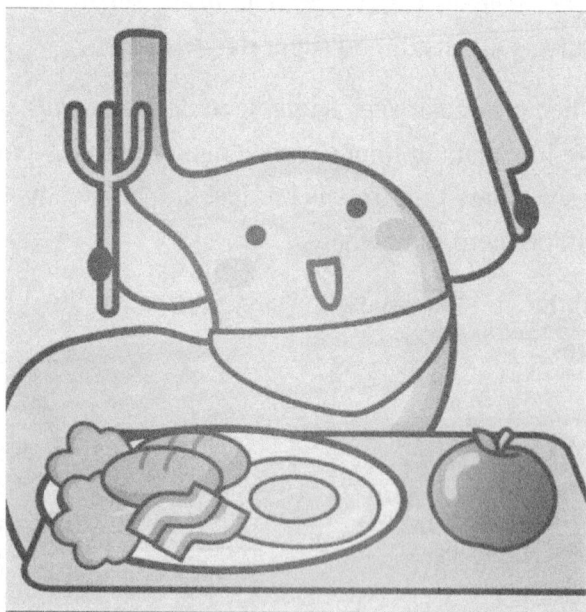

'All the things that sugar helps with can be shown to help with digestive function. And all the things that help with digestive function can be shown to help with everything that sugar helps with, so where you begin isn't the most important thing, as long as sugar is involved.' Moi

When it comes to health, looking at ways to improve digestion is a great place to begin. That's because it is central to so many problems. But it's also because it is reasonably quickly experimented with and usually relatively easy to see if the experiments work.

Digestive issues are often an early sign that something needs to be corrected. For example, when stress goes up, most people notice an impact on digestion, one way or another. More and more, science proves that severe illness is related to digestive dysfunction, which isn't coincidental.

If you have any health issues, it's logical to look at what is happening in the digestive system or do things to help improve digestion. Laxatives have a long history of treating illnesses, including severe diseases like cancer.

It makes sense to limit food intake when an issue impacts digestive function. Many people are attracted to fasting to improve health or treat illness. There are reasons why that makes sense. But only up to a point.

Luckily you don't have to throw the sugar out with the bathwater. You might be surprised to learn that most of what you get told about sugar is the opposite of the truth.

If you want to know the truth about sugar, just read as many things as possible about the harm that sugar causes and then flip it on its head. It's a great way to discover what sugar can help prevent or heal.

And the truth about sugar is that it is great for digestion, which means it is excellent for metabolism. So now that you know that sugar restriction causes stress and blood sugar dysregulation, it should be no surprise that it promotes digestive issues. But conversely, digestive issues promote stress and blood sugar dysregulation. And then it's no surprise sugar gets blamed for all this. Unfairly.

Chapter 18 / The Problem With Fasting>>

Fasting can be beneficial. Not eating food when stress or illness interferes with digestion can help reduce the intestinal issues that drive disease. It makes sense to reduce the load on the digestive system and hopefully remove stress placed upon the liver, allowing it to function better. That will likely play a significant part in recovery, no matter the issue.

But unfortunately (or fortunately), our system functions slightly differently than, say, a car. You can't just wash out the pipes, and off you go. Of course, you can only do that with a car sometimes, but you get my point.

After fasting (sometimes briefly), glycogen (backup sugar) stores will deplete. Cortisol levels will go up as part of a process for providing energy via the conversion of protein into fuel. The stress from the fast also increases the release of free fatty acids, as another way to provide the fuel required by the body. A rise in the release of fat into the bloodstream, more so when composed of large quantities of PUFAs, directly inhibits thyroid hormone activity and interferes with glucose uptake by the cell.

A large portion of inactive thyroid hormone (T4) conversion into metabolically active thyroid hormone (T3) occurs in the liver. It requires glucose to be able to enter the liver cells effectively. Fat accumulation in the liver can inhibit this process.

A thyroid deficiency directly interferes with the storage and release of glycogen in the liver, which means less readily available fuel and, therefore, more stress substance release. So, as you might be starting to realise, this can become a circular downward spiralling situation.

People use fasting to improve metabolic function. But lack of fuel (as well as protein and other nutrients) means more stress, which means interference with metabolism, including interference with the ability of the liver to do what it does to help with recovery.

When it comes to detoxing, good liver function is crucial. The liver plays a significant role in preparing toxic substances for excretion (glucuronidation) to protect vital organ systems (including the brain) from unnecessary, damaging exposure. Unfortunately, the more toxins in circulation – including bacterial endotoxin and breakdown products of PUFAs – the harder it is for the liver to do its job.

So, in other words, you don't want the thing you do to take the stress away from the liver to be the thing that also puts more stress on the liver. That's especially true when you consider that you need the liver to function better, to fix all the things that interfere with liver function. Confusing?

It doesn't have to be. Let me word it another way. Suppose the method recommended to clean the system to improve health interferes with the function of one of the primary cleansing organs. In that case, you should be suspicious.

It is not controversial from a biological point of view. When the liver operates sub-optimally, metabolism is compromised, and vice versa. Interference with thyroid function is at the top of this list of things that interfere with liver function.

And stress is at the top of the list of thyroid-inhibiting things. So you cannot withdraw sugar from the conversation or the damage done by PUFAs. The stress from a fast increases the release of free fatty acids, directly interfering with the proper use of sugar. That means suppressed thyroid and liver function and reduced detoxification capability. There's no magical way to get around it apart from fueling your system with sugar.

The breakdown products of PUFAs promote oxidative stress. Oxidative stress is a central factor in liver disease, including NAFLD. Also, PUFAs encourage insulin resistance, which is involved in the progression of many metabolic illnesses that fasting gets used to try to help, including liver disease. Unfortunately, fasting can increase exposure to all of this.

To add fuel to the fire, running out of fuel, increasing stress, and suppressing thyroid metabolism also interfere with digestion and intestinal barrier function. And the digestive system and intestinal barrier are crucial for protection against toxins. As digestion slows, bacteria tend to multiply, and this eventually causes an increase in the release of bacterial endotoxin. More endotoxin causes a rise in serotonin, estrogen, nitric oxide, and other stress substances in the intestines and (because of the reduction in gut barrier function) also throughout the system.

The substances of stress can directly injure the liver and further suppress metabolism, making the situation worse than it originally was. When more bacterial toxins pass through to the liver and the rest of the system, it increases stress, inflammation and blood sugar dysregulation. It means more exposure to PUFAs and more interference with liver function.

Endotoxin reduction is one of the initial benefits of fasting, and that is a legitimate benefit. The problem is, however, that it can backfire depending on the particular conditions.

Another benefit of a fast is avoiding PUFAs and other metabolically interfering ingredients in food. It can lead to an overall reduction in digestive system toxicity and detox load. That is until it leads to increased release of PUFAs into circulation. It can be tricky.

So yes, even though fasting does benefit some people some of the time (there will always be people who swear by it), it isn't the panacea it's said to be.

One of the liver's jobs is detoxifying estrogen so it can get excreted via the digestive system. However, excess estrogen prevents the liver from doing this job properly and interferes with metabolism inhibiting thyroid function. It can add weight to the potential downward-spiralling nature of things.

Suppose a fast has the effect of slowing thyroid metabolism and digestion. In that case, this can interfere with producing hormones like progesterone that oppose estrogen, worsening estrogen dominance issues. People often fast to improve health issues driven by excess estrogen and decreased progesterone. It needs consideration.

So one big problem with fasting is that metabolic conditions vary. Unfortunately, the people who need help the most and who use fasting to fix more severe issues can potentially get the worst results.

However, they can occasionally be lucky if they quickly recognise that there are better ideas than fasting.

Others, perhaps with more metabolic resilience, only become aware of their damage once they have been doing it long enough. But guess what. There are ways to get around this to get the benefits of fasting without the negative aspects.

Chapter 19 / The Art Of Fasting, Without Fasting>>

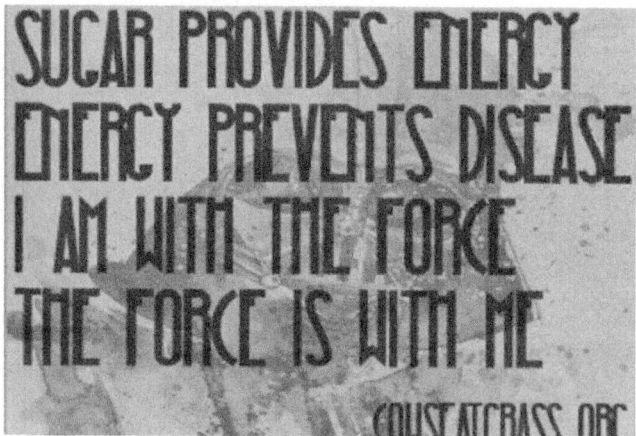

SUCAR PROVIDES ENERGY
ENERGY PREVENTS DISEASE
I AM WITH THE FORCE
THE FORCE IS WITH ME

FOUSTATCRASS ORC

Suppose you want to get the benefits of fasting without really fasting. Or in other words, without the downsides. In that case, this is what you need to do. You need to provide fuel to keep stress at bay without fueling bacterial issues in the intestines and without adding an unnecessary workload on the liver. Simple.

The easiest way to achieve that is by using an easily assimilable fuel source to replenish and maintain glycogen stores, providing a continuous fuel supply. You provide the fuel necessary to help energise the liver and allow it to do its job (especially concerning detoxification and support of thyroid metabolism). In addition, it helps protect against rising stress and inflammation, enabling recovery from illness. And guess what the most accessible and assimilable fuel source is available in this universe? That's right, sugar.

Am I saying all you need to eat is white sugar, and you will be healthy? No, I'm not, but you already knew that. And if you didn't, it might have something to do with not having enough sugar available. So it's OK; I forgive you.

Contrary to all the popular anti-sugar hype, simple white sugar is biologically proven to be a metabolism-enhancing, liver-energising, thyroid-promoting substance.

Sugar is the perfect fuel for the liver. The fructose component in white sugar or sucrose powerfully stimulates glycogen storage. And you convert any excess sugar not burned (usually much less than imagined because of the metabolism-stimulating effect of sugar) into anti-inflammatory and protective fats. As mentioned earlier, this can also help improve metabolic health conditions.

Because you can convert excess sugar into triglycerides – as protective fats for storage in the tissues – it is far less of an issue (if at all) than excessive fat consumption. That's because the fat consumed almost always has a component of PUFAs. So it ends up causing interference and damage to the metabolism.

Is excess consumption of sugar the cause of fatty liver? It's a popular belief, but the evidence points to the things that interfere with the use of sugar. As stated earlier, most things, like polyunsaturated free fatty acids, are increased due to stress, sugar avoidance, and fat consumption. So at the very least, it's not that black and white. And suppose excess sugar gets converted into fat. In that case, this has more to do with metabolic suppression than anything particularly fattening about sugar per se. It's more accurate to see sugar as something that increases the number of calories used, and as such, as something that eventually helps to regulate fat stores properly.

Other things also play a role in helping the liver and metabolism function. For example, protein intake and specific vitamins and minerals sometimes need to be considered to improve results when using sugar therapeutically. But when it comes to getting the most out of protein and other nutrients, it is essential to get enough sugar. Otherwise, you can end up wasting your nutrition and increasing stress. Depending on the condition of your metabolism, sugar-to-protein ratios required to reduce stress and improve thyroid function can vary significantly. Some people do well with a 2:1 sugar-to-protein ratio; others need as much as 5:1 or even higher.

The best way to work out what works best for you is by experimenting and seeing what happens concerning things like anxiety, digestion, and sleep. Learning how to measure thyroid function is fundamental. Besides looking at symptoms of suppressed thyroid, methods include tracking pulse and temperature changes, CO_2 monitoring and Achilles heel reflex.

People fast to improve digestion, but sugar promotes digestion in various ways. The digestive system requires fuel to function optimally, and it also requires proper thyroid function and proper liver function.

So by improving thyroid and liver function with sugar, you are improving digestion. And limiting digestive issues helps protect the liver, enhances the thyroid, and so on. Improving digestion, liver function, and thyroid metabolism helps lower exposure to inflammatory stress substances (like estrogen, serotonin, nitric oxide, and endotoxin). However, these increase when sugar levels are low, and all interfere with thyroid energy metabolism performance.

Simple white sugar is straightforward to digest and reduces bacteria's ability to grow in various ways. White sugar is directly anti-bacterial but also in many indirect ways. For example, increasing thyroid energy metabolism is anti-bacterial. It is not a made-up theory. Hypothyroidism is a significant driver of small intestinal bacterial overgrowth (SIBO).

And guess what. White sugar improves the function of insulin by improving thyroid, digestion, and liver function. It does all this by lowering stress, inflammation, adrenaline, cortisol, etc., and limiting exposure to polyunsaturated free fatty acids. You probably don't hear that every day. But that doesn't mean it isn't true. You can quickly check it out for yourself.

On top of that, even without that reduced stress effect, white sugar is far less insulinogenic than many other carbohydrate sources.

Chapter 20 / Improving Digestion Improves Everything>>

There isn't a disease in the world not connected to digestive function one way or another because our system functions as a whole, not as a bunch of separate independent parts.

But the digestive system is fundamental because it's where we put our food, hoping that it gets used to assist with the functioning of the whole system. And as the digestive system gets compromised, getting the most out of our food becomes harder and harder.

Suppose the food we eat is a problem in the beginning. In that case, that alone can be the thing that interferes with digestion. Even if it gets digested, it can interfere with other systems that interfere with digestion. So if the food is a problem and digestion is compromised, you can see how that can be a big issue.

It's all interconnected, so an unhealthy mind can also impact digestive function. Still, poor digestion can affect the state of mind. There are many simple biological explanations as to why this is the case.

Most people know the direct link between mental and emotional stress and digestion from experience.

Whichever way you look at it, improving digestion helps with all other systems. As mentioned earlier, improving digestive function reduces exposure to stress and inflammation-promoting substances, including endotoxin, cortisol, adrenaline, nitric oxide, estrogen, serotonin and PUFAs.

Rising levels of the substances of stress promote disease and inflammation in general, and it isn't difficult to find evidence of the truth of this statement. No condition isn't known to worsen with increased exposure to stress and stress-substance release. For example, rising cortisol, estrogen, lactic acid and nitric oxide, and the breakdown products of PUFAs, promote cancer growth and spread.

And every disease is connected to issues with digestion. So healing is more likely if you reduce exposure to things that cause digestive distress, even if it's just for short periods. That's because we already have a self-healing system. It's just that it has to be allowed to function. And interference with digestion interferes with function.

But it isn't always easy because the things that promote digestive distress accumulate in the system over time and get released into circulation under stress conditions. So it can feel like a puzzle.

You want to get the things that interfere with metabolism out of your system. Still, you release them into circulation to get them out of your system. Then they go about causing more harm.

It is especially true when restrictive diets get used, trying to avoid toxins and remove them from the system. But unfortunately, the restriction is itself a form of stress. So it increases exposure to stress substances while simultaneously releasing fat and toxins into circulation. It is the worst combination, the main reason dieting often fails and worsens metabolism.

There is no perfect solution to this problem because life doesn't work that way, and neither does metabolism. However, improving metabolism improves the ability to remove toxins from the system safely. So if there is a perfect way to solve this issue, this is it. You let metabolism do what metabolism does as best as possible.

You want to figure out ways to avoid toxins, reduce stress, and improve metabolism, improving digestion. And you want to do it gradually because that is the safest way. And the primary method is to ensure that the metabolism continues to get fueled and that it can use the fuel it is getting. The best kind of fuel to ensure that is sugar. You can't just rely on sugar and nothing else, but sugar is what you need one way or another. It isn't sugar's fault if the metabolism can't use the sugar you give it. Once you stop blaming sugar, you can start to figure out where the stumbling blocks are. Often the stumbling blocks are the toxins consumed and the stress-promoting things released. And they can't all be avoided, especially not straight away.

So there are no guaranteed immediate results because problems that take time to develop also take time to fix. Anything is possible, however. One thing guaranteed is that improving digestion and liver function and lowering overall metabolic stress is a good idea, no matter what.

Section D / Why Quitting Sugar Feels Good

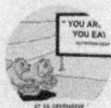

> **CowsEatGrass**
> @CowsEatGrassBlg
>
> Did you know, sugar is 980 times more addicting than misery.
> #sciencefiction
>
> 10:13 am · 20/11/19 · Twitter for iPhone
>
> ┊ View Tweet activity

'The thing about giving preference to sugar restriction is that it can – at least at first – feel pretty good.'
DanM@CowsEatGrass

One of the biggest problems with quitting sugar is that it can initially make you feel good. "What's wrong with that?" you ask. I'll tell you.

Chapter 21 / Sugar Isn't The Junk In Food>>

'It isn't sugar that's the problem with "junk food". Sugar isn't the problem with any foods, not anywhere.' CowsEatGrass

When people decide to quit sugar and get healthy, the first thing they often do is remove what they consider to be junk food from their diet. But unfortunately, it's popular to refer to these foods as "high-sugar foods".

Not long after they stop eating these foods, they start to feel good, which locks in the idea that sugar makes them sick, and quitting sugar has made them feel better. But there's a problem with that conclusion.

Most of the time, if you discover more detail, you quickly realise that sugar is the last thing you quit. You will often find that foods labelled as high in sugar are high in a long list of harmful ingredients. So again, PUFAs are possibly the number one culprit, even though there is a lot of competition for first place.

The things that get quit include harmful gums, heavy metals, preservatives, flavour enhancers, and other things that have no place inside the food. You also quit wheat glucose, other starches, and maybe some simple white sugar.

But because junk foods get lumped together and referred to as "high-sugar foods", and they repeat the lie often, it is accepted and hardly ever questioned. But, of course, there is nothing wrong with quitting harmful ingredients. It's an excellent idea.

The problem that arises is a problem of mistaken identity leading to wrongful conviction. There are also harmful ingredients (for example, PUFAs again) in the so-called health foods that then get eaten as a replacement for the so-called junk foods. As a result, the good feeling only sometimes lasts. What happens next?

What tends to happen as a result of this error in the

identification of ingredients is that it leads to people thinking they need to quit sugar even more than they already have. Then they again disregard the importance of avoiding the real culprits.

Sorry to say, this can once more lead to a person feeling good for a while, further cementing the belief that quitting sugar is the way to go. "What's the reason now?" you ask. The reason is that stress can feel good until it doesn't.

Chapter 22 / Stress Can Feel Good, For a While>>

If you quit sugar enough, your body will compensate by increasing stress hormones like cortisol and adrenaline to provide fuel from the breakdown of tissues and the release of fat into the bloodstream.

Yes, it's true. Releasing stress hormones can make you feel good temporarily, and I have nothing against people feeling good. The problem is that the good feeling only lasts for a while. The longer you expose a person to higher than optimal levels of cortisol and adrenaline, the more it can cause harm to metabolism, eventually leading to anything but feeling good.

But before that happens (it can take a while), a person can get attached to the idea that quitting sugar is responsible for their most significant health improvement. It can be tough to let go of the belief.

This misconception is extremely powerful and is responsible for a great deal of confusion and, eventually, lots of unnecessary pain and suffering.

People often remember feeling a sense of euphoria, and frequently problems that they have struggled to fix for years miraculously disappear.

Energy levels can improve, digestion can improve, mood can improve, skin can improve, and even sleep can improve. But it doesn't last, and there is more than one reason.

For starters quitting sugar and raising stress is a little like taking a drug that makes all your problems disappear and makes you feel great. It's a lot like that because the kind of drugs I'm referring to work by raising cortisol and other stress substances. You probably know that if you do it for long enough, the good feeling starts to wear off, and your problems worsen.

The logical explanation is that the stress substances are part of an emergency backup system. Ideally, you want to avoid emergencies, although if you can't avoid them and you have to rely on stress substances, they will keep you going. It could be better, but it's better than the alternative.

Contrarily, it doesn't make sense to continuously put your system in an emergency state to get the benefits from raised stress. But that is what quitting sugar is all about. It's like setting fire to the house so you can get the help of your sprinkler system. It sounds silly when you say that, but it's a valid comparison. Luckily, the system slows down if the stress continues for too long. It either happens sooner or later.

So chronically increased exposure to stress eventually suppresses metabolic function, ultimately worsening the areas that get a boost from the powerful effects of the stress substances. So now you have damage from stress and damage from metabolic suppression.

Suppressed thyroid slows digestion, which promotes bacterial issues. Suppressed metabolism also interferes with gut barrier function, allowing more toxins into the primary system. Increased bacteria leads to the release of endotoxin, which now passes through to the liver, placing the liver under more stress.

A stressed liver cannot carry out detoxification and thyroid hormone and cholesterol provision. And thyroid hormone and cholesterol play a significant role in protection against stress and inflammation. Endotoxin is directly inflammatory, and inflammation promotes disease. Cholesterol protects against endotoxin.

And this is just the beginning. Stress, thyroid dysfunction, and digestive distress promote excess exposure to estrogen, nitric oxide, serotonin, lactic acid, and other potentially harmful stress substances, including releasing PUFAs from storage.

So what starts as a feel-good scenario can lead to a cocktail of metabolic interference. Some good things can come out of quitting sugar. But the reason is more complicated than "sugar bad."

It doesn't always happen overnight, but sugar restriction leads to metabolic interference if you go for long enough. And the longer you quit sugar, the harder it is to reintroduce sugar into the diet. That's especially true if you don't know what's going on and how to avoid the mistakes that made you want to quit sugar in the first place. So for something reasonably simple to explain, it can be complicated.

Chapter 23 /
Hibernation is Not a
Lifestyle Choice>>

The temporary suppression of metabolism from stress exposure is good because it protects against more immediate severe outcomes.

For instance, it can temporarily protect against vitamin and mineral deficiencies, and it can protect against a too-rapid breakdown of valuable muscle and other tissue.

I'm not against that. It is one reason we can survive through starvation and other hardships.

For this reason, it is always a good idea to start slow when bringing sugar back. Sugar is powerful. So if your system is trying to protect itself from a lack of nutrition, it's wise not to give it too much fuel too quickly.

And suppose metabolism has been under stress for

a long time. In that case, large quantities of stress-promoting things might still circulate in the system. So putting your foot down on the pedal too rapidly can increase stress. It is one reason why people can gain weight when they start eating sugar again after being on a low-carb diet. But, of course, it is not sugar's fault; it usually also involves other ingredients, so the details matter.

The purpose of this book is not to say sugar is magic; eat more, and everything will be fine. If that were the case, I would say that. But it isn't the case, although it is closer to the truth than suggesting that sugar causes disease and you should quit eating it.

So yes, slowing metabolism by eating less sugar can have unintended benefits for people with nutritional deficiencies and other metabolic issues. Still, the benefits will not last for the same reason that animals do not hibernate forever. They know better.

It's a defence mechanism, not a lifestyle choice. When the circumstances change, and what they need becomes available again, out they come. And what those things are for humans, at least, include sugar—sometimes called carbohydrates.

But not all carbohydrates are made equal. For

example, some kinds of carbohydrates can be more challenging regarding digestion and their impact on blood sugar stability. But not the kind most people think.

Chapter 24 / Not All Sugar Gets Made Equal>>

Quitting some kinds of sugar can, at least until a person is better able to handle it, be a good idea.

But it isn't the first kind of sugar most people try to get out of their diet. It isn't the evil white sugar or even the evil fructose that everybody fears.

I'm talking about the complex carbohydrates people get told to have 650 servings of every day.

These carbohydrates are supposed to be slow-release but increase blood sugar and promote insulin far more than plain old white sugar.

That's because they get converted into pure glucose, which is released more quickly into the bloodstream and increases insulin far more. Shocking, I know.

Also, the complex carbs tend to get filled with

difficult-to-digest fibres, anti-nutrients, and PUFAs that can interfere with the digestion and assimilation of nutrients.

Complex carbs are recommended for their fibre content because it gets said that this makes them digest more slowly. In a way, it is true, but it is misleading. They often have allergens, even carcinogenic substances, which interfere with digestion. And fibres found in foods like beans and cereal grains can irritate the intestines and feed bacterial issues. Increased exposure to bacterial endotoxin promotes blood sugar dysregulation. But, once again, it gets blamed on the sugar content of the food.

There is good reason to think that excessive cereal grains and starch intake can promote bacterial issues, inflammation, thyroid dysfunction, and blood sugar dysregulation. But it is far more likely when combined with a diet high in PUFAs. If anything, the combination of PUFAs and starchy hard-to-digest carbs, rather than sugar per se, can be responsible for problems mistakenly blamed on white sugar.

For these and other reasons, complex carbs can be a problem for metabolism, and quitting them, at least temporarily, can be beneficial.

It leads to confusion around the idea of quitting sugar. Nobody in their right mind stops eating healthy complex carbs and consumes more diabetes-causing "evil white sugar", the so-called toxic fruit sugar. Well, almost nobody, anyway.

So the first thing you need to ask when a person says they quit sugar and feel so much better is, what do you mean when you say "sugar"?

Are you referring to the sugar found in fruit, or are you referring to some form of starch or plain glucose? Or do you have all the different kinds of sugars grouped in your mind as if they were one thing? Or even worse, do you mean food with some variety of sugar and 654 other ingredients that all get a free pass?

Just that information can make a big difference to what you think happens when you consume "sugar" and help you untangle the confusion.

Section E / How To Use Sugar Therapeutically

SUCROSE

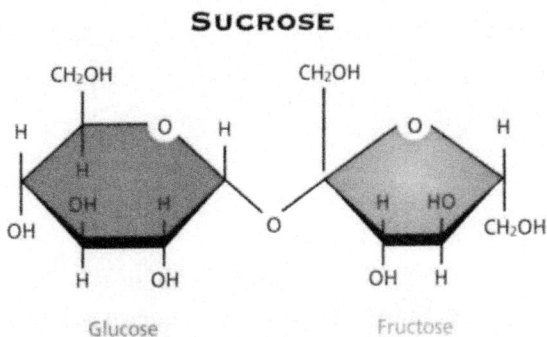

CH₂OH · · · CH₂OH

Glucose · Fructose

SO SWEET!

'Knowing how to use sugar is the easy part. The hard part is knowing why you can trust that sugar is good for you and then actually trusting it.'
Me@CowsEatGrass

Congratulations! You made it. Hopefully, you now realise that there are significant scientific and logical explanations for why sugar is good for you. And you may also be starting to let go of some of the fear associated with sugar.

It takes time to disentangle all of the propaganda and bad arguments because, whether you realise it or not, you get constantly exposed to anti-sugar rhetoric. Once you start to see it, you will see it everywhere. And once you free yourself, you will never be able to be caught in the net again. Rarely anyway.

As soon as you understand how sugar gets mistakenly blamed for disease, even in scientific studies, it will become much more difficult to fool you.

Now it's time to talk about how sugar can be therapy. There isn't just one way to use sugar therapeutically. That's because sugar can be therapy no matter how you use it, with a few obvious exceptions.

So I will talk about how I have used sugar over the years that have helped me and others I know. And then, you can decide for yourself what you think will work best for you and go from there.

Everybody's needs are individual, at least to a certain extent. I haven't had any bad experiences with sugar, per se. Not that I know, anyway. Nor do I know anybody else who has.

When it comes to sugar, ever since I realised the power it had over a decade ago, I've been pushing the envelope. So you never know. I may hit maximum intake eventually.

Chapter 25 / Simple Sugar Syrup>>

I use sugar therapeutically. One way is by dissolving as many teaspoons of white sugar as I need at a particular time with a tiny bit of water to make it into syrup.

I do the same thing more often with a tiny bit of milk or orange juice. Just enough to make it into a syrupy drink but not enough to make it into a regular drink. Roughly about a quarter of a cup. I do this at night if I wake up, have trouble relaxing or falling back asleep, and don't want too much liquid in my belly.

Sometimes I will do something similar briefly before I do something stressful, like exercise. It is because I want energy without too much digestive stress. And this explains one of the main reasons white sugar is uniquely therapeutic. It provides the energy to protect against stress in a way that does not create much work for digestion.

It is crucial, mainly when conditions are stressful, for instance, when you are about to do something that will put extra strain on your body or mind. And the same principle applies when bringing down stress in a compromised system. In other words, a metabolism that is under a lot of stress.

That's what therapy is all about—dealing with suboptimal conditions. The fact that some people do not require any help (so I've heard) does not detract from the importance of therapy.

I have found that the number of teaspoons of sugar per shot of syrup that works best depends on circumstances like the stress levels you face. It also depends on the condition of your metabolism. For example, if you improve thyroid function and increase the ability of the liver to store glycogen. In that case, going for more extended periods is possible without replenishing glycogen stores.

It works for a couple of reasons. Firstly there is less stress, so there is less need for sugar. Secondly, the liver can store more sugar so you can go longer without more.

I can't say how much is the right amount for you, although I can say that I have experimented with a wide range of amounts per shot and day. It depends on many factors and differs from person to person and daily. It doesn't have to be precise. A guess will usually do; your instincts will improve over time, and you will learn to adapt to changing conditions.

Once again, I am not saying you can survive on white sugar alone. Metabolism needs more than just fuel. However, it is crucial. I'm not a doctor or health professional; this is not medical or nutritional advice. However, you should consult your health professional before deciding what to do with nutritional therapy. Especially when it comes to something as risky and addictive as white sugar, right?

Chapter 26 / Sugar Added To Drinks>>

The second most common way I use sugar therapeutically is to add white sugar to my daily drinks. I will most commonly add sugar to coffee, milk, and orange juice. It keeps my blood sugar more stable throughout the day, replenishing glycogen stores and reducing stress.

I first experimented with sugar as therapy when my system was very stressed. At that time, smaller amounts of sugar at more regular intervals throughout the day were an effective way to go about it.

I also found that as time passed, it became easier to replenish glycogen and the longer I could go without having sugar or other food. Not that I would go for that long. Not often, anyway. But you get a sense that your blood sugar and metabolism are stabilising.

You can explain this in several ways. Mostly it is

because the more you keep stress at bay, the less exposure you have to the things that interfere with liver function and glycogen storage. The lower the stress, and the better liver functions, the more glycogen you can store and the less glycogen you go through.

Using sugar for therapy is intended to get you to a point where you no longer need treatment. Then you can use sugar for energy when you need it simply because you like it. It is food.

When you first use sugar as therapy, with high stress and low glycogen stores, smaller amounts more regularly make sense to me. Not that it's the only way, but it's a fast way to improve. Removing PUFAs from your diet and out of tissue storage is very important, as are some other nutritional requirements.

However, as a general rule, keeping stress down and improving blood sugar supply and stability improves overall metabolic efficiency. You don't necessarily need to eat large amounts of sugar to get the therapeutic benefits of sugar. Instead, using small amounts more regularly can effectively keep stress at bay and blood sugar stable. It is especially relevant for those with lots of PUFAs stored in tissue and who have issues with weight gain. Small amounts of sugar more regularly can go a long way towards reducing free fatty acid exposure. The release of PUFAs into the bloodstream under stress interferes significantly with metabolism and prevents PUFAs from being removed safely.

Stress makes me more inclined toward anxiety and metabolism "running too fast". As a result, I found, especially early on, that it sometimes required more sugar in one go to get the desired results. So I always combine my drinks with a pinch of salt and get calcium, potassium, and magnesium from milk, OJ, and coffee. A healthy metabolism requires alkaline minerals, but a suppressed metabolism wastes the alkaline minerals. It is difficult to say what individual requirements are. Like sugar, some need more than others. Measuring metabolism, for example, by tracking pulse and temperature changes, is an effective way to determine individual needs.

It is worth mentioning that coffee has many proven therapeutic benefits, especially concerning liver function. As I said in one of my articles on coffee, 'Coffee For MS – Wonderful!' (in the 'The Anti-Inflammatory Fantasies Folio' eBook), coffee works best with sugar. It is especially true when a person has stress-related metabolic issues.

Coffee stimulates metabolism powerfully. When people with metabolic issues consume too much coffee without enough sugar, it promotes a stress state, increasing adrenaline and other stress substances. They might then miss out on some potential benefits of regular coffee consumption. But coffee heals liver function and improves metabolism over time.

Depending on what I want, I often have multiple teaspoons of sugar in my drinks throughout the day. And I rarely have a coffee with less than five teaspoons of sugar, and often more. That's just how I roll.

I don't know what will work for others. And, once again, this is not medical or nutritional advice, as I am not qualified to hand that out. Nor does it serve you to be told what to eat or how much to have. Check with your friendly health professional before making any health-related decisions.

Chapter 27 / When I Have Sugar>>

I have sugar at many different times throughout the day. Still, I will always have sugar (if possible) before and after I do something stressful, as in something that requires more than average energy. Nothing complicated to understand about that, but it is surprising how many people will do something stressful, like exercise, for example, first thing in the morning without replenishing sugar stores.

It's good to exercise on an empty stomach because exercise suppresses digestion and intestinal barrier function, exposing you to bacteria and endotoxin and causing many problems. But you want to practice the art of having an empty stomach without being devoid of glycogen stores. That is what sugar therapy is all about—using sugar to manipulate metabolic circumstances in your favour. It is not about evolution or ancestral diets;

it's about helping deal with the stress of life.

First thing in the morning, I usually have OJ with sugar and some milk and sugar, followed by coffee with sugar. Then, throughout the day, I have sugar in my coffee, OJ, or any other drink I might have. And, of course, I have natural foods and beverages with sugar, like rice or potatoes or food with added sugar, like cola, which I love.

As I mentioned before, I will use sugar to help bring nighttime stress down if necessary, either as I'm going to bed or if I wake up or both. But, again, I might do this multiple times on some occasions if necessary.

Suppose I ever feel like I'm coming down with something. In that case, I will usually simplify my diet to the bare basics, sometimes just OJ and sugar (sometimes with a pinch of salt), coffee with milk and sugar, and cola. It is another situation where the art of having an empty stomach without running out of fuel can be beneficial. Again this is not medical or health advice, just some things I have experimented with over the years that I have found very helpful.

There is no one correct answer to metabolism and health. My book, 'The Feeling Overrides Nutrition', discusses how tension in the mind-body and mental and emotional stress can override nutritional therapy. This book is about understanding how and why sugar can be helpful. Then the application part can take on many different forms. The most important principle is that stress makes digestion more complicated, and stress is an insufficient energy problem. Sugar can help limit mental and emotional stress, and stress reduction can amplify the benefits of sugar.

It's essential to remember that an attempt to meet stress with "energy" intake has to consider how difficult or easy it is to use what you consume for energy. So it can be helpful to add simple white sugar into something easy to digest with other potentially beneficial stress-reducing nutrients, like OJ.

Often OJ isn't optimally ripe, so added sugar can replicate riper juice, at least to a degree. And it can potentially help protect against irritation caused by less than perfectly ripe juice.

Chapter 28 / How Much Sugar To Use>>

How much do you need, and how much is too much sugar? The answer to this question is that it depends. It depends on levels of stress and the state of metabolism, the condition of the liver, and the digestive system. These things are all interrelated.

It also depends on how much PUFAs and other inflammatory things you have stored in tissue. It depends on nervous system condition and levels of biochemical stress and inflammation throughout the body. And it depends on the availability of protective substances like progesterone and testosterone. Tracking symptoms, pulse, and temperature can be helpful again because it indicates how metabolism functions.

But as far as I'm aware, there's no one magic answer to the question of how much, and yet there's a long list of helpful possible solutions. So it would be best to research the subject and experiment to determine what works for you.

Some people use (and need) more sugar than others. Some can only deal with smaller amounts initially, gradually increasing intake as metabolism improves. It is far more common that less than what is needed gets consumed rather than more than is required to get results.

But yes, sometimes small amounts of sugar more regularly are enough to do the job. I'm unaware of any fixed rule except that removing sugar from the diet isn't the solution.

You can get your sugar in a variety of different ways. Still, I probably wouldn't use lots of white sugar as therapy, for long periods, without also getting the nutrients needed to go along with it. That said, I've never found it too difficult to get what I believe are sufficient nutrients from OJ and milk and a few other things, even with more and more white sugar.

Or, to put it another way, I haven't noticed vitamin and mineral requirements changing significantly, as I have more sugar. But results may vary.

Still, lowering stress and inflammation, especially with sugar and avoiding PUFAs, reduces the wastage of nutrients more than it increases nutrient requirements. However, a minimum will still be necessary. There are scientific studies that point towards this conclusion.

Remember that when more sugar is consumed in one go than the metabolism can handle, it increases lactic acid. It generally does not feel good. So having less at once makes sense under these circumstances until stress reduces and energy metabolism improves. However, as stated earlier, quitting sugar altogether is not an effective way to reduce stress and enhance metabolism. So it does not solve the issue of excess lactic acid either.

The only way to fix the ability of metabolism to deal with stress is to do so with the inclusion of sugar. To some degree, anything else is using stress to deal with stress. And that is stressful.

Chapter 29 / Sugar On Wounds>>

'Gather round for a story about wounds and the evil things that prevent proper healing. It's the same old tale of woe with all the usual suspects. Stress, low thyroid, inflammation, bacterial endotoxin, serotonin and PUFAs are named. Sugar, the legendary hero, comes to the rescue again.' Sugar Heals Wounds, CowsEatGrass.org

In my article 'Sugar Heals Wounds' (in my eBook 'The How To Hasten Healing Handbook'), I explain in detail (including lots of studies) how simple white sugar helps heal even serious wounds. It also includes so-called "untreatable" diabetic ulcers, of all things. I have used white sugar on my wounds for a decade and found it very effective.

I have found that pure icing sugar (fine powder) is helpful because I can pack it into wounds without irritating tissue. Then it stays on and dissolves into the damage. Some people like to make a paste out of sugar and water. Using icing sugar usually makes that unnecessary. I have also used white sugar topically on burns.

Keep in mind that there are good reasons why the consumption of sugar also improves healing. It makes sense once you understand that sugar doesn't cause diabetes but can help heal it and why people with diabetes have issues with wound healing.

Exposure to too much stress interferes most with the wound-healing process. And the most critical question is, What interferes with the availability of energy needed to deal with the additional stress of a wound? Unsurprisingly, stress is more challenging when thyroid energy metabolism is already impaired. Wounds are no exception.

PUFAs are released from storage into the bloodstream when blood sugar runs low under stress. The breakdown products of PUFAs interfere with proper wound healing and promote a chronic inflammatory energy system impaired state, which inhibits effective healing.

Also, rising bacterial endotoxin exposure, high cortisol levels, and excessive secretion of serotonin, nitric oxide, and estrogen (all substances involved in the progression of the diabetic state, cancer, and heart disease) prevent proper wound healing. The high lactic acid in wounds is a marker for chronicity, and CO_2 therapy (as well as thyroid hormone application) has successfully treated chronic ulcers and other serious injuries. There are other interfering factors. However, the pro-thyroid pro-CO_2 anti-stress influence of sugar consumption and topical sugar application makes sense as part of a safe and effective wound healing regime.

Once you discover sugar heals wounds, if you want to believe sugar causes disease, you must also think very confusing and contradictory things. For starters, you must think sugar causes diabetes, and diabetes causes non-healing wounds and diabetic ulcers. And that you can heal these wounds and ulcers with topical sugar. Hmm.

Section F /
Diseases Not
Caused By Sugar

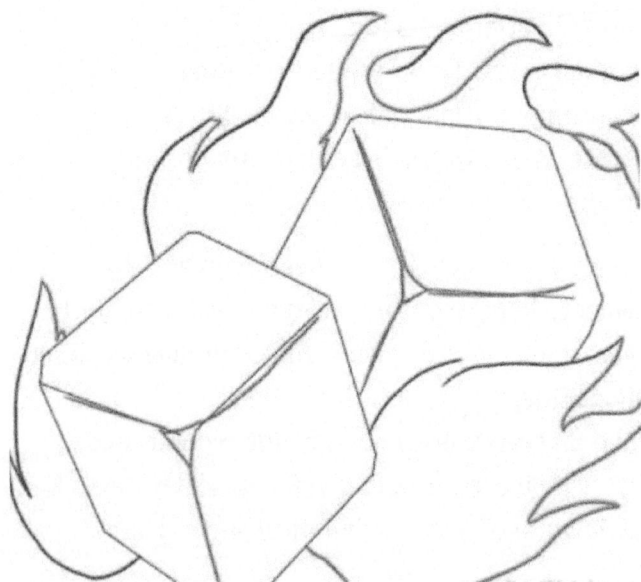

'Everything bad you ever heard about sugar is true, about lack of sugar.'
CowsEatGrass

'The mainstream narrative requires you to believe that sugar causes diabetes, diabetes causes problems with wound healing, and topical sugar heals wounds, but that's just some strange paradox.' I said that.

'The one thing sugar does best is not cause disease.' Anonymous, or was it me?

Here are a few diseases not caused by sugar. Not a comprehensive list because sugar does not cause any disease. Unless, of course, you do not allow sugar to do its job. And then sugar still does not cause disease.

Chapter 30 / Autism and Sugar>>

'When stress rises, and you inhibit thyroid function, digestion is directly affected. And you don't need to look very far to find out that digestive issues always go together with autism, and this is not just some weird coincidence.' CowsEatGrass

Just quickly search the internet, and you will find an endless supply of articles claiming sugar worsens autism. Does it? In my article 'The Autism Metabolism' (in 'The Autism Arthritis AIDS Alzheimer's Anxiety Almanac'), I discuss what science demonstrates is associated with autism symptoms.

Hypothyroidism, inflammation, intestinal distress, endotoxin and oxidative stress get mentioned. Also included are lipid peroxidation, high cortisol, serotonin, nitric oxide, lactate, low cholesterol and iron accumulation.

Based on the above list and the information in Section A of this book, it's easy to see sugar doesn't cause or worsen the things that promote autism symptoms. Instead, the opposite is likely to be true.

Stress, or lack of sugar availability, increases cortisol, adrenaline and lactic acid, releasing PUFAs from storage. PUFAs promote thyroid and cholesterol issues and interact with excess iron. The result can be inflammation, slow digestion and digestive distress, plus increased bacterial endotoxin, serotonin, and nitric oxide. And that's just one way of looking at it. The potential configurations are endless.

That does not mean that the foods that most people think of when they talk about high sugar intake don't make autism symptoms worse. Unfortunately, those foods usually combine starch and PUFAs, with a few ingredients possibly made by NASA (I'm joking) thrown in at no extra charge.

Ask a few questions about what the person in question eats. It usually doesn't take long to find some stress-promoting, thyroid-suppressing, digestion-interfering, inflammatory culprits.

Chronic emotional stress is also a significant factor in autism and a primary driver of digestion-related issues. And it's essential to remember that chronic digestion-related problems, combined with inflammatory things mentioned and known to be involved with autism, also promote emotional distress.

It's a circular issue, and many approaches can be highly effective. Still, it helps to know the truth about how things work together. And the truth is sugar is always involved in disease because sugar is central to metabolic function. So the problem is not sugar per se; the problem is what is interfering with sugar metabolism. That is a significant factor involved in every disease. Autism is no exception.

Suppose you believe sugar is bad for you. In that case, it becomes much easier to convince you that the stressful things that promote autism are helpful. And that makes things very confusing and challenging.

Chapter 31 / Cancer and Sugar>>

'The idea that sugar feeds cancer is prevalent and has recently been heavily promoted. As a result, many believe it would be wise to remove sugar from the diet altogether.' Sugar Feeds Cancer, CowsEatGrass

We all know sugar feeds cancer, right? Well, not exactly. Sugar fuels all cells, but cancer will eat everything, especially fat and protein.

I go into detail about this in my previous writing (including 'Sugar Feeds Thyroid' in 'The Stress Less Digest' and 'The Anti-Cancer Articles eBook') and provide lots of science showing what feeds the growth and progression of cancer. But scientific studies aside, it's also illogical to think that something as crucial to metabolic function as sugar could be behind cancer.

Especially if you also think that exposure to too much stress can cause cancer. Or if you believe that chronic inflammation can make cancer get worse. Or that interference with energy metabolism function can be something that promotes the growth and spread of cancer.

That's why it makes sense that PUFAs can be a significant factor in cancer progression. For starters, it's easy to confirm that PUFAs (including the storage of PUFAs in tissue) have increased far more than any increase in white sugar consumption over the last few decades. And it's easy to find information about what the PUFAs are known to break down into once inside your body. After that, it doesn't take much to discover that these breakdown products of circulating PUFAs are a significant driver of stress, inflammation, and cancer.

The idea that sugar causes pancreatic diseases is prevalent. But it is unscientific and unsubstantiated. The breakdown products of PUFAs (like MDA and 4-HNE) promote oxidative stress. Oxidative stress increases inflammation. And inflammation and oxidative stress drive the progression of pancreatitis. Chronic pancreatitis is well known to be an essential factor in the development of pancreatic cancer.

Once you know about the thyroid-suppressing, inflammation-promoting breakdown products of the PUFAs (including seed oils and fish oil), you can look into other things that promote cancer. High cortisol, nitric oxide, lactate, serotonin, and estrogen are significant. Also relevant are low cholesterol and iron dysregulation. These are all things that happen under stress, inflammation, and excess exposure to PUFAs.

Chronic stress, or anything that interferes with thyroid energy metabolism and digestive function, increases bacterial issues, causing more significant exposure to bacterial endotoxin. Endotoxin is a powerful independent promoter of inflammation. And exposure to PUFAs suppresses metabolism and digestion and interacts with circulating bacterial endotoxin. The inflammatory effects of PUFAs and endotoxin are synergistic. They encourage pancreatitis and the onset and metastasis of cancer of the pancreas.

Bacterial endotoxin exposure directly promotes an increase in the release of serotonin. Serotonin plays a role in developing pancreatitis and many kinds of cancer. Stress, PUFAs, inflammation, metabolic suppression, and endotoxin exposure also increase nitric oxide, interfering with energy metabolism and further promoting stress and inflammation. In addition, increasing systemic levels of nitric oxide are involved in the growth and spread of cancer, including pancreatic cancer.

After that, all you need to do is remember that stress uses up sugar. When sugar isn't available, everything mentioned above can happen more. In particular, the release of PUFAs into circulation. And once you know that all the stressful inflammatory things promote each other and make it harder to use available sugar, lightbulbs should go off.

People are recommending ketogenic diets as a means to prevent and treat cancer. But increased ketone production in the body occurs under conditions of metabolic stress (or starvation), which fuels the growth and metastasis of cancerous tumours.

Cancer cells are known to undergo metabolic reprogramming to make available the energy required for rapid growth and proliferation. When sugar levels diminish, cancer cells adapt by shifting their metabolism toward ketone and fatty acid oxidation. For example, the requirements for advancing malignant gliomas come from sources other than sugar. Fatty acid oxidation is a critical component of brain tumour metabolism. And ketogenic diets increase fatty acid availability, which the tumour utilises.

Many other things can promote cancer, including inflammatory gums, heavy metals (not just iron), radiation, and more. Either way, sugar should probably be starting to sound more innocent.

Based on what sugar can do concerning stress, there are many good reasons to start believing that sugar is highly protective and therapeutic, even with cancer.

Chapter 32 / Diabetes and Sugar>>

'It's an understatement to say many recommend sugar restriction to improve health. Still, evidence indicates that this approach is potentially unsafe and can become a powerful driver of worsening inflammation and disease.' Me

Practically everybody in the world thinks that sugar causes diabetes. And yet, once upon a time, people used sugar to treat and cure diabetes effectively. So why are people so sure it causes it? The most obvious reason is the misleading conflation of blood sugar dysregulation issues with sugar consumption.

And once you look at biology, what causes blood sugar dysregulation is apparent. Eating white sugar isn't high on the list. Are you surprised? Or are you shocked? Or both?

I was amazed when I searched through all the published studies on diabetes, insulin resistance, and related issues. I kept finding out more about the breakdown products of the PUFAs and bacterial endotoxin, cortisol, nitric oxide, lactic acid, inflammation, and of course, the subject of stress in general.

The incredible thing is that taking sugar out of the diet can cause all the things that aren't caused by eating sugar per se. For example, this includes chronically high blood sugar. And many things can increase blood sugar, but not all are harmful. Thyroid hormone is one example.

And chronic hyperglycemia – a symptom of metabolic dysfunction – can be alleviated with more significant amounts of sucrose or fruit sugar in the diet rather than by its avoidance. But, of course, I'm not saying the only thing wrong when someone has problems properly regulating blood sugar is that they aren't eating enough sugar.

But it isn't helpful to talk about sugar dysregulation issues in a simplistic sugar-blaming manner. It helps to look at stress's impact on proper metabolic function. Moreover, the assumption that high blood sugar or hyperglycemia drives the diabetic state is also inaccurate. Elevated lactic acid is strongly associated with type 2 diabetes due to decreased oxidative capacity. And stress interferes with oxidative ability. The breakdown products of PUFAs interfere with the use of sugar. They are closely associated with the progression and severity of symptoms of type 2 diabetes.

Also, adrenaline and cortisol promote insulin resistance, encouraging blood sugar dysregulation and other metabolic issues. And everybody knows stress elevates adrenaline and cortisol.

Sugar lowers stress and all the other things on the list of thyroid metabolism-related issues. Gradually removing the PUFAs works very well with all this. So can some other stuff, like smiling, relaxing, and not worrying too much.

But back to sugar. You can't take sugar out of the picture. As I have said many times in many different ways, as soon as you stop eating it, your body will start turning you into sugar, and when it does that for too long, it comes with a very high price.

Chapter 33 / Heart Disease and Sugar>>

'You'd think with all the guidelines and advice about heart health; hearts would be getting stronger, healthier and happier. But no, in "upside down world", you might have to think again.'
DanM@CowsEatGrass

The idea that sugar causes heart disease is another widespread misunderstanding. This one is a bit more complex because many myths are associated with high cholesterol and what is said to drive it.

And then there's the whole eating cholesterol/saturated fat causes heart disease mantra. My book 'The Thyroid, Cholesterol, Happy Heart eBook' details this subject. I have concluded that, much like sugar, concerning heart disease, science does not find what most people think it finds.

But lots of good science does show that many things caused by stress and inflammation and suppressed thyroid energy metabolism cause heart disease-related issues. And, of course, the breakdown products of PUFAs are actually at the heart of this story.

So are thyroid dysfunction, digestive distress, intestinal barrier dysfunction and excess endotoxin. And serotonin, nitric oxide, lactic acid, cortisol, adrenaline, iron dysregulation, and more.

The traditional diet-heart hypothesis says lowering serum cholesterol by replacing saturated fat with PUFAs will slow the progression of atherosclerosis and improve survival. But there needs to be more clarity regarding the role of cholesterol. And regarding what happens when you lower it by interfering with the ability to produce it.

Chronic inflammation and biochemical stress drive heart disease. For example, as a defensive response, cholesterol levels tend to increase under stressful inflammatory conditions. Cholesterol gets used to produce protective substances, including pregnenolone, testosterone, progesterone and DHEA. And proper thyroid function is also crucial to their ongoing supply. These substances are protective against stress and inflammation, and heart disease.

Because the breakdown products of PUFAs interfere with the ability to produce cholesterol, damage cholesterol and suppress thyroid function and energy metabolism, they interfere with natural protection against inflammation. Saturated fats, however, have many anti-inflammatory protective effects. Sugar promotes cholesterol production and metabolism, as well as the production of progesterone and other protective substances. Plus, excess sugar can get turned into saturated fat.

Energy needs to get made available for the heart to function correctly under stress; not all ways are equal. Therefore, over time, exposure to less-than-optimal energy provision methods can change the structure and function of the heart.

When stress is high, and sugar availability is interfered with, thyroid system function gets suppressed. It causes the heart to get more easily tired when it needs to work harder than usual. As a result, defensive stress processes get activated. Fat gets released out of storage to provide an alternate energy supply.

Today, these fats are often highly polyunsaturated

in composition, and the byproducts of the PUFAs powerfully suppress thyroid performance and promote inflammation, interfering with and damaging the heart.

When heart cells get damaged by a lack of energy and increased exposure to the breakdown products of the PUFAs, you need sugar for healthy cellular regeneration. But unfortunately, sugar is prevented (by the fat released) from being used by the cells.

Lack of sugar availability also increases adrenaline (and other catecholamines) and cortisol, which further interferes with the use of sugar, encouraging exposure to PUFAs, and preventing optimal heart function.

As part of this worsening stress scenario, lactic acid gets produced in more significant quantities. High lactic acid is another factor involved in suppressing thyroid system function and promoting heart failure.

A stressed, hypothyroid, inflamed heart exposed to increased lactic acid can become increasingly fibrotic, further hindering heart function. Conversely, increasing thyroid function, thereby lowering lactic acid (and promoting CO_2 production), can reverse fibrosis in the heart, allowing the muscle to regenerate and enabling improved function.

There is more to say about this, including the role played by increased exposure to estrogen and serotonin. You can't necessarily eat more sugar and automatically fix these issues. Still, sugar is protective and therapeutic in everything known to damage heart function/metabolic performance.

Chapter 34 / Obesity and Sugar>>

'Calories matter to weight loss but only relatively speaking. Metabolism is where the real magic happens. A "fast" metabolism is driven either by the thyroid or stress. It's easy to see both as the same...but they aren't.' CowsEatGrass.org

Another thing not caused by eating sugar is everybody's favourite one for blaming sugar. That is obesity. I am six feet tall. I weigh 80kg (give or take 1 or 2 depending on minor fluctuations). My weight has mostly stayed the same over the last ten years, no matter how much sugar I add to my food or swallow. But forget about me for a moment. Maybe I'm an outlier. I may have a fast thyroid metabolism. (Which is the point, isn't it?)

Regardless, I can tell you I'm not the only one. I know many other people who use sugar therapeutically who aren't obese or gaining excessive weight. But even that isn't a convincing argument. But "the science", I hear you say. What does science say?

For starters, you must get through all the junk science that does things like using questionnaires to find out what 50,000 people ate over the last 30 years. And then they completely disregard all the things that cause obesity and zoom in on any sugar found. That's if the people questioned even remember or tell the truth when answering questions.

Then there are the studies that find stress and blood sugar issues in the results and blame eating sugar in the discussion and conclusions. So what is going on there?

And then there's the science that finds one thing and gets interpreted entirely inaccurately in articles talking about the results of the science. So there's any number of things that can be going on there.

And finally, there's actual biology performed reasonably well and hopefully honestly. Of course, you can never be 100 per cent certain of that, but you get a knack for being able to tell the more time you spend analysing studies. And I have spent quite a lot of time doing that, I can tell you that much.

And can you guess what most excellent quality studies find behind obesity? If you said thyroid energy suppression, inflammation, stress, the breakdown products of the PUFAs, cortisol, serotonin, endotoxin, estrogen, nitric oxide, lactic acid, etc., guess what? You're right.

Other factors are involved. You can't just eat sugar and automatically solve all issues relating to weight gain. And it is common to hear people talk about how they gained weight when they reintroduced sugar into their diet. There are valid explanations, and none of them is that there is something uniquely fattening about sugar. The truth is closer to the opposite. But if your metabolism is exposed to a lot of stress and is not functioning as well as it can, adding sugar back into the diet in large amounts too quickly can cause weight gain.

Stress can keep the weight down, and reintroducing sugar can bring it down, increasing weight. Alternatively, other metabolic issues (including various nutritional deficiencies) can interfere with the ability to use sugar. That can also lead to weight gain. It's best to explore these things. After years of stress and interference, it can take time and experimentation to improve metabolism.

But although it can be tempting to think that rapidly losing weight by quitting sugar and doing all sorts of other stressful things comes without a cost, it doesn't. It is common to see rapid ageing, and often the weight gets put on again after the urge to eat sugar gets too intense. Now the body composition and metabolism are in a worse condition. What is required is a better understanding of what is interfering with metabolism, consistent changes, and patience. It is not easy, and success is not guaranteed.

And obesity doesn't happen in isolation from other metabolic issues just because you ate some sugar. So it's no coincidence that obesity and diabetes and cancer, and a long list of other diseases often go together? Obesity is a defence mechanism, as is the disease process in general. It would be best to respect that before you "attack" it.

But once you realise that you have been blaming sugar unfairly again, you are one step away from learning how sugar can be a therapy. For almost anything you imagine me saying. Yes, that is what

I am saying. But, at the very least, it's a mind-blowingly long list.

Section G / Sugar For Stress

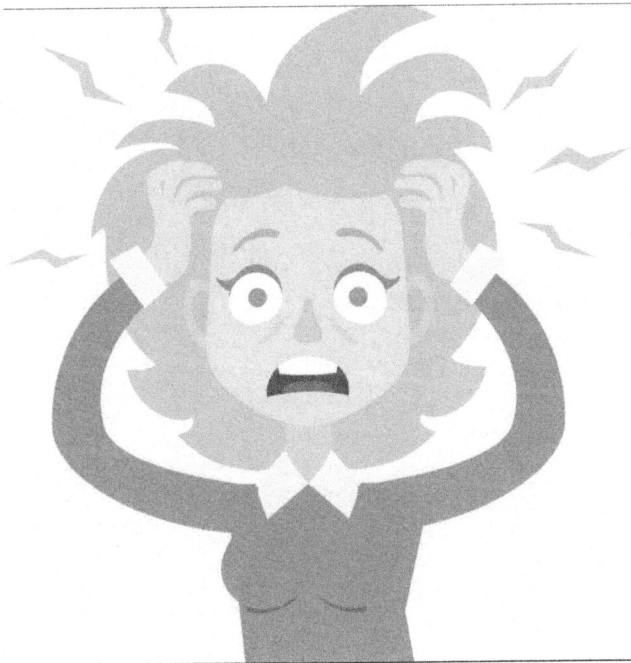

'The most stress-promoting thing about sugar is not having enough of it, especially when you're stressed.' Says I

Chapter 35 / Stress Increases Sugar Needs>>

This book is about the relationship between sugar and stress. Everything I have mentioned up until now relates to one or the other. Or both.

Lack of sugar isn't the only thing that causes stress, and sugar isn't the only solution to problems with stress, but the two are uniquely tied together. Biologically speaking, excess stress is known to be an energy-deficient state, and sugar is our primary source of energy. Of course, you can dispute that, but I have yet to hear an objection that holds up to logic, reason, or biology. Not that that's enough to stop people from trying.

Yes, there are other things involved in the process. But keeping things simple, either you can meet stress with sugar (energy), or you cannot meet stress with sugar (energy). At some point, you have to eat sugar, or else you are meeting stress with stress. And that's stressful. Again, that's in line with biology.

Sugar isn't the only ingredient determining whether or not it is possible to handle stress effectively. Still, consuming sugar is one of the most fundamental ways to help improve the whole range of things that happen biologically that result from excessive stress exposure. That includes increased sugar needs.

Of course, you have to keep in mind that stress can also interfere with the ability of metabolism to use sugar properly. It is part of why sugar often gets a bad name. And it is also why it isn't always possible to fix stress-related issues simply by eating more sugar. And I indeed never suggested it is always possible.

It helps to consider other things when trying to improve your sugar metabolism and protect against stress. I will tell you some of those things in the next chapter, but first, it's essential to be clear about something.

Yes, eating sugar is not necessarily enough to fix all metabolic issues. And yes, overeating sugar can add to problems when metabolism is damaged. But that doesn't mean quitting sugar as a solution makes sense. The problem is you have an increased need for sugar because of stress, but stress is getting in the way of using sugar properly. So what to do?

You want to avoid undersupply of sugar because it creates stress. But you also don't want to overload your system with sugar if all it does is more of the same. Luckily there are good ways to look at this situation, and it doesn't have to be complicated.

Chapter 36 / Eating Sugar Versus Making Sugar>>

Overeating sugar will almost always be less of a problem than not eating enough sugar. That's because when you don't eat enough sugar, the stress-related things in your body get magnified because not having enough sugar is stressful. That sounds like a circular argument, but that's because we're talking about a circular problem.

Controlling how your metabolism responds is challenging if you don't eat enough sugar. It will, however, react by doing what it does to turn parts of your body into sugar. Making sugar is a primary survival response.

High cortisol and adrenaline are often the first things, followed by an increased free fatty acid release that interferes with sugar metabolism. It can then lead to digestive issues, which raise bacterial endotoxin, promoting inflammation and the release of serotonin. Then there can be a rise in estrogen, nitric oxide, lactic acid, histamine, etc. After that, who knows where it ends?

Often thyroid metabolism will slow down to protect against the catabolic effects of rising stress. But this comes with a price, especially over the long term. And the payment is generally with increased ageing, degeneration and disease.

On the other hand, if you eat more sugar than you can handle, you might convert too much of it into lactic acid rather than carbon dioxide. That isn't a good thing to encourage, but it's pretty easy to tell when it's happening because it won't feel good. But there are ways to combat it. Reducing the quantity of sugar consumed in one go is the obvious first thing to try.

Spreading sugar intake can help keep blood sugar stable and stress down. That (as well as a smaller amount eaten in one go) will increase the likelihood that you will use the sugar more efficiently. Then over time, the overall metabolic function will have a more significant opportunity to improve, allowing for more sugar in one go with no adverse consequences.

But what about hyperglycemia, I hear you say?

Well, that does not get caused by sugar per se. It is caused by eating more sugar than the body can metabolise, caused by stress and metabolic interference. I've already explained that, but it's also worth mentioning that you can have hyperglycemia without overeating sugar. You can have hyperglycemia eating no sugar at all. Stress causes hyperglycemia, and not eating sugar increases stress. So which is worse, hyperglycemia from eating sugar or making sugar? Well, you know my answer. The one that comes with more metabolic stress is worse.

Several vitamins, minerals, and other things also help lower stress and optimise the ability to utilise sugar. For example, biotin, thiamine, niacinamide, glycine, taurine, coffee and activated charcoal are beneficial. Also, aspirin, minocycline, famotidine, cyproheptadine, and methylene blue can help. Enough salt, magnesium, calcium and potassium can also be crucial for stress and blood sugar regulation.

The whole concept of "overeating sugar" is misleading. It is not something that happens in isolation. Sugar is naturally in foods with other ingredients and gets eaten with other ingredients. And so, it can be challenging to work out what is causing the issues. Then if you try to remove sugar to see if it's causing the problem, that comes with many complications I discussed earlier.

Many people have experimented with making sugar to improve health and metabolism, which always backfires. The experiment that rarely gets carried out is seeing what happens when you no longer expose sugar metabolism to many interfering things. Yet, that is the most rewarding experiment. But it takes time to improve, and the damage doesn't all disappear in one go. Healing is not linear. But one thing is sure: eating sugar needs to be involved and can be very therapeutic.

Section H / How and Why They Blame Sugar

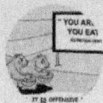

CowsEatGrass
@CowsEatGrassBlg

I just stopped eating 648 different ingredients. I feel so much better...now that I've quit sugar.
#sciencefiction
12/9/18, 4:56 pm

ılı View Tweet activity

'There must be a reason sugar gets blamed for health problems. But, of course, it can't all be a mistake, can it? Well, come to think of it, there are some explanations. The problem is that sugar being the cause of disease, isn't one of them.' CowsEatGrass.org

Chapter 37 / Sugar Is The Perfect Scapegoat>>

Sugar makes a great fall guy if you're unaware of (or want to hide) the genuine causes of disease.

Suppose you want to sell products filled with cheap and easy ingredients, and you want to divert attention away from the fact that the components are harmful. In that case, it helps to have a patsy.

Suppose you want to be able to blame something for the diseases caused by harmful ingredients in your products. In that case, it makes sense to blame something almost impossible to avoid. Something that we need and crave. Something that our body immediately starts turning itself into if we run out for even a second. Something like sugar.

Sugar is in most tasty foods. Of course, it's not the

only thing that makes food delicious, but it's big.

Chances are you have sugar in your diet. But even if you don't, there's always the sugar being made inside you to hold responsible and keep the blaming narrative going. "You must be accidentally or secretly eating sugar", they'll say.

Then those same people who profit most from harmful ingredients will also say, "get rid of more sugar from your diet, and you won't be in this situation!" But you will be in this situation even more so.

If only sugar weren't so crucial to the functioning of your system, you'd be fine. But the truth is you will never be able to get rid of sugar well enough. And that's precisely the way they like it.

Chapter 38 / Blood Sugar Dysregulation>>

The most common way sugar is blamed unfairly for causing disease is by incorrectly conflating blood sugar dysregulation with sugar consumption. Nothing could be further from the truth. And yet people are conditioned to assume issues with blood sugar result from overeating sugar.

It isn't something people think about much at all. You might as well be talking about the colour of the sky. Everybody knows it's blue, and that's as far as it usually goes. Similarly, everybody knows sugar causes blood sugar dysregulation issues. Right?

No. But everybody thinks it, though. You can't know things that aren't true. You can only believe them. And it isn't true. Looking through the biological evidence, it takes little time to notice that various things cause blood sugar dysregulation.

Unfortunately (or fortunately), eating sugar isn't one of them. Not eating enough sugar can more accurately be understood as a cause of blood sugar problems. I discuss this in detail in Section B of this book. I also discuss it in my articles and eBooks (particularly 'The Better Blood Sugar Balancing eBook'), which include many scientific studies as additional evidence.

But if you've gotten this far, you are probably starting to realise that what I am saying here makes sense, even without the studies.

Unfortunately, many people are never made aware of this. So it's easy to lead them astray simply by telling them that sugar causes blood sugar issues. It could be intentional or by accident, but it isn't accurate either way.

Chapter 39 /
Distraction From The
Issues>>

Blaming sugar for almost everything helps to take attention away from many things that cause many problems. But unfortunately, the people promoting the harmful products get to call them "health foods" and make vast amounts of money while people get sick. So I prefer to call them "hellth foods".

And they say, "Hey, it's the sugar!" So then you think you need less of that and more of the things that make you unwell. So fish oil and other PUFAs are the first things that come to mind, but there are many other things.

It gets very confusing, mainly because most people don't quit sugar altogether, so they never get to find out how bad an idea it is. And even when they do stop sugar enough, it can take time to figure out that it's a bad idea because quitting sugar can feel pretty good for a while. And it's always hard to eliminate the lingering doubt, especially since the whole world is waiting to tell you how evil sugar is.

And the "right way" isn't easy. Because so many things promote stress, and not just food ingredients, removing one of them only sometimes leads to immediate recovery. As I said earlier, recovery isn't linear, and it can take time to heal what took time to cause. So there's lots of opportunity along the way to doubt whether sugar is that innocent after all.

Chapter 40 / You Need Sugar>>

If people who make money from selling you unnecessary things find a way to ensure you don't feel well, there's a long list of things they can get you to do and buy to try and feel a bit better.

That sounds cynical or even far-fetched, but imagine how much money gets spent on treatments or therapies, not to mention retail therapy, to feel better.

The higher the stress, the more money is spent. It takes little mental gymnastics to see that some people will benefit significantly if the population's stress increases.

And the great thing is that it doesn't stop the sale of sugar, just in case they make money out of that, too, because, at the very least, people will keep bingeing on it whenever the urge gets too intense.

Thankfully, the urge doesn't completely disappear

because I don't need to tell you what would happen if it did. But you know what I'd say by now.

Chapter 41 / Your Brain Needs Sugar>>

Your brain is the organ that needs the most sugar. So not getting enough sugar can make your brain function suboptimally, especially in the face of stress. In addition, the more people cannot use their brains properly, the easier it is to manipulate them.

Call me a tin foil hat-wearing conspiracy nut if you like. Still, influential people worldwide can influence information and benefit significantly from manipulating the population more efficiently. It sounds shocking, but you know it's probably true.

And guess what? Once you convince people that sugar is harmful, making them avoid it, keeping them convinced sugar is unhealthy becomes easier. But only because it isn't if you understand what I mean. If you don't, you might need more sugar.

Chapter 42 / Lack of Sugar Slows Metabolism>>

Because when sugar runs low, stress increases, removing sugar from the diet can, at least in the short term, make a person feel better. Stress hormones can do that short-term, but it's not all roses.

It is not good to have chronically raised stress hormones; over time, they can less make you feel better and become part of what makes you sick.

When stress increases and energy availability decreases, metabolism slows down to protect you. It is one way people feel better, and symptoms can temporarily abate. It's suitable for survival but not necessarily for long-term health.

It explains why you can make people believe that sugar is the problem. The reason is that it's a matter of context. And sugar is involved with metabolic problems because sugar is involved with everything to do with metabolism. So it's a case of guilt by association.

Chapter 43 / Nutritional Deficiencies Make Sugar Look Bad>>

It is easy to get enough vitamins and minerals if you can access things like milk, seafood, liver, etc. Still, it's worth remembering that speeding up your metabolism too quickly can make nutritional deficiencies more noticeable.

That's not to say that sugar causes nutritional deficiency, as it is popular to believe. What it is is that you need other nutrients in your diet, and you can't live on sugar alone.

Vitamins and minerals can also play a part in hindering or improving the ability to metabolise sugar properly, but the opposite is also true.

That is, sugar helps with the proper use of minerals

and vitamins. That's not to say it wastes them; stress can do that, but sugar protects against stress and protects against nutrient wastage or dysregulation.

But yes, pumping up metabolism too quickly can be an issue when there is a need for certain other vital nutrients. But again, that isn't the fault of sugar per se. "Follow the stress" or "follow the malnutrition" might be another way of looking at it.

Chapter 44 / Metabolic Issues Make Sugar Look Bad>>

Metabolic dysfunction includes liver issues, blood sugar instability, and high levels of PUFAs in circulation. And various other things are interfering with the ability of the cell to use sugar. So it makes sugar look bad.

It's wise to take things slowly to heal from years and years of stress and chronic sugar restriction, especially when reintroducing sugar into your diet. And you don't want to move too quickly and give the anti-sugar movement more excuses to accuse sugar wrongly, do you?

But remember that stress and lack of sugar availability or accessibility caused the issues first, so don't start thinking this is another excuse to quit sugar.

The irony is that you need sugar to fix the issues preventing you from using sugar to fix the problems you need sugar to avoid. Does that make sense? It does to me.

So sugar helps with the things that promote stress and blood sugar-related issues. Included are thyroid dysfunction, digestion and liver issues, exposure to PUFAs and other harmful inflammatory things, and general stress and metabolic dysfunction.

Chapter 45 / Bad Ingredients Make Sugar Look Bad>>

It's easy to blame sugar for disease when so many food ingredients (many of which aren't food at all) cause harm to metabolism. It's like blaming the house's walls for the fire after throwing gasoline all over them and then setting them alight.

Highly unstable fats, heavy metals, inflammatory gums, flavour enhancers and several other things that have no place in any food are a recipe for disaster. These and some other things interfere with metabolic function, making sugar look like the problem. But what's wrong is that you can only get some of the benefits of the sugar you eat.

Again, that doesn't mean quitting sugar under these circumstances will improve anything. Maybe temporarily, it's possible, but is that a solution? Unfortunately, no, and the longer it goes, as mentioned many times, the worse things get.

Eventually, the floodgates open and, well, put it this way, you don't want to experience a crashed metabolism. It can take years to recover fully. I know many people who can vouch for that.

Chapter 46 / Bad Science Blames Sugar>>

Minus the application of the scientific method, science isn't science. Even when applied, the scientific method is not foolproof, but much of science today is far from scientific. It's more like science fiction. And the more you examine studies about sugar, the easier it becomes to see that often, they are fiction, not science at all.

Sometimes studies make claims that aren't proven, and they often refer to other studies that make claims that aren't proven. So how do they get away with it? The meta-analysis is an excellent example of big claims that often don't add up. You have to review the individual studies to see things clearer. But who does that?

Some studies find something good about sugar or bad about something else, yet still conclude that sugar is the problem. Go figure. Yes, sometimes it can be a case of genuinely different opinions and interpretations or unintended bias; perhaps it's even dishonesty.

I'm not saying I am the ultimate authority on the validity of scientific findings. Still, the more you read studies that find or imply bad things about sugar, the more you will see that what I am saying here is valid.

Chapter 47 / "High Sugar Foods" That Aren't>>

It's always funny to see the foods called "High Sugar Foods" these days and to realise that they are primarily high in almost anything but plain old white sugar.

Most of the time, the culprits are high in PUFAs, starch, fibres, and a long list of things possibly invented by NASA (I'm joking again). Then maybe there's a tiny little bit of sugar in the food. And guess what it's called. I'll give you a clue; it's not called "High In Everything But Sugar Food".

And yes, they throw the orange juice and cola under the bus with all the doughnuts, mass-produced pizzas, etc.

It becomes one big confusing mess, so it's not a wonder nobody knows what to believe. But on the other hand, confusing people can be an intentional tactic.

Chapter 48 / Different Kinds Of Sugar Have Different Effects>>

Not all sugar is made equal. For example, suppose a person has blood sugar-related metabolic problems. In that case, too many starches or pure glucose consumption can exacerbate issues.

Again, this is especially true when consumed with PUFAs and other harmful ingredients, so it isn't as black and white as some think.

Suppose people struggle to digest a baked potato mixed with salt and butter. In that case, plain old white sugar or sucrose (and foods high in sucrose and fructose) can still be therapeutic.

However, the opposite gets repeated in the "anti-sugar upside down world".

Chapter 49 / Sugar Raises Insulin>>

One of the most common ways sugar gets blamed for a disease is by repeating the prevalent mantra, which states that sugar raises insulin levels. Of course, everybody knows insulin issues are a significant factor causing illness. However, several things could get improved with this widespread belief.

First, plenty of evidence shows that excessive stress and inflammation due to too much exposure to the PUFAs and their breakdown products and endotoxin causes insulin dysfunction. High cortisol and adrenaline can promote insulin resistance, as do the stress substances serotonin, estrogen, lactic acid and nitric oxide.

On top of all that, many things can increase insulin, including protein, but sugar (sucrose and fructose) lowers exposure to stress and helps improve insulin function. Just eating more sugar isn't the solution every time. You have to be able to metabolise it, but you already know that.

Foods filled with starch or glucose, like bread, rice, and cereal grains, are far more insulinogenic than simple white sugar. However, most people think the opposite is true.

Again, it's an unintentional error, but there may be some unintended financial benefits for people not interested in setting the record straight. Coincidentally, of course.

Section I / How To Use This Book

Your brain needs sugar to function optimally...if you don't understand this, you probably need sugar.

CowsEatGrass.org

This book is not a diet book or instructional manual of any kind. It is not health advice or any other sort of advice, for that matter.

Step-by-step guidelines can help up to a point. Still, life is complicated, and more than one thing is usually responsible for causing any problem. For this reason, it often takes more than one change to fix a problem. Not always, but most often.

However, certain things are easily changed and can lead to significant improvements. Changing the way you understand and use sugar is a big one. This book is about sugar, but it isn't only about sugar.

You can use the information provided here to work out how to include all sorts of foods therapeutically, as well as many non-diet-related treatment methodologies and other lifestyle changes.

The interconnected nature of things in the mind-body can help you improve health and well-being without necessarily knowing what's causing what is wrong. But, of course, there is almost always more than one issue anyway.

And there are no guarantees because life is full of mysteries beyond my pay grade to understand or explain. So please don't take anything in this book as a prescription or advice manual for salvation or longevity. Instead, I hope the information will help you feel better and get more enjoyment out of life.

But also remember, some of my views have changed over the years. For example, I was almost a vegan once upon a time. So who knows, I might even be a "breatharian" one day.

Why are there no references provided in this book, you ask? Here are a few reasons:

1. You can find thousands of references to published peer-reviewed studies in my articles and eBooks, available for purchase at cowseatgrass.org.

2. You can find almost all the references you need for free on PubMed. Put any of the claims made in this book into a search engine and add the word PubMed, and you will find studies. An example of one search might be 'diabetes endotoxin PubMed'. Or call endotoxin by its other name, lipopolysaccharide. Or change it to 'LPS insulin resistance PubMed', etc.

Sometimes you have to be more tricky, especially if you're looking for studies on the harmful effects of PUFAs. Try searching with the name of one of the breakdown products of PUFAs, like malondialdehyde or acrolein. It isn't hard once you get the hang of it.

3. This book is intended to help you understand how sugar is healthy. It isn't another book that adds a long list of studies that get disregarded with the claim that studies are dishonest or faulty. And yes, often that is true.

4. Even though I have learned a lot from reading studies, scientific studies often won't change a person's mind. It would help to hear accurate explanations before being motivated to look for and read many complicated studies. I got a lot of motivation from the work of Dr Ray Peat. With the understanding I gained from his work, I found the studies to back it up.

5. There will always be studies that back your position, and there will always be studies that go against it. Before you can decipher between them, it helps to understand some of the bigger picture biological principles.

I recently published another book, 'The Feeling Overrides Nutrition', looking at alternative ways to understand and deal with the problem of excessive stress. It doesn't include studies. And I liked to sip on cola while I wrote it.

Thank you for reading, and I wish you the best of luck, good health, and lots of smiles, laughs, and happiness. They are one of the best things for metabolism, especially combined with sugar.

Printed in Great Britain
by Amazon